ESSENTIALS
of
FINANCE
in
NURSING

Barbara A. Mark, RN, PhD
Assistant Dean for Research
and Program Development
School of Nursing
Medical College of Virginia
Virginia Commonwealth University

Howard L. Smith, PhD
Professor
Anderson Schools of Management
University of New Mexico

AN ASPEN PUBLICATION®
Aspen Publishers, Inc.
1987

Rockville, Maryland
Royal Tunbridge Wells

Library of Congress Cataloging-in-Publication Data

Mark, Barbara A.
Essentials of finance in nursing.

Bibliography: p.
Includes Index.
1. Nursing services—Business management. I Smith,
Howard L. II. Title.
RT86.7.M37   1987   362.1'73'0681   86-28780
ISBN: 0-87189-614-1

Editorial Services: Ruth Bloom

Library of Congress Catalog Card Number: -
ISBN: 0–87189–614-1

Printed in the United States of America

1 2 3 4 5

To my parents, Marion and Jack, the teachers, and to my sister, Judi, the listener.

Barbara A. Mark

To my family and friends.

Howard L. Smith

Table of Contents

Preface

Essentials of Finance in Nursing was written to help nursing administrators understand basic financial management concepts and the financial functions of health care organizations. It is intended to provide an introductory understanding about the financial environment of nursing and health care institutions. This text should help nursing administrators to analyze financial reports and statements, financial performance, sources of revenue and costs, and debt structure. In addition, it should assist them in managing current operations while considering the broader financial issues and context of their organizations. Emphasis is placed on explaining the financial and capital needs of health care organizations. All of the above is taken from a nursing perspective.

This book is intended to help nurses and nursing administrators understand the financial requirements and operations of their institutions. A related purpose is to help them participate more effectively with other managers and staff members. The book is not designed to make nurses into financial managers, nor is it designed to be the sole source of information for financial concepts. *Essentials of Finance in Nursing* sets a foundation from which nurses and nursing administrators can build a knowledge base. Supplemented with experience and further study into sophisticated use of these basic concepts, it should help them to make a more effective contribution to nursing program, department, and organizational performance.

Essentials of Finance in Nursing can be used by nurses who have never previously read a financial management text. However, those who have will find that the text places financial concepts into a comprehensive outlook with specific application to nursing. Consequently, it can be recommended to several audiences. This book should be useful in degree-oriented nursing courses, continuing education seminars, and self study.

Acknowledgments

The authors would like to acknowledge the support of the School of Nursing at the Medical College of Virginia/Virginia Commonwealth University, and the Anderson Schools of Management at the University of New Mexico in the preparation of this text. Special thanks is also extended to Barbara Brown and Marie Wood for their help in typing the manuscript.

Chapter 1

The Financial Management Context

Nursing administrators have long been responsible for providing safe, effective nursing care in health care institutions. Yet the extraordinary changes that have occurred in the hospital industry over the past decade have given rise to new demands and challenges.[1,2] As a result, nursing administrators are increasingly involved in strategic decisions that have an impact on institutional adaptation and long-term survival.[3,4] Poulin's recent study of the role of today's nurse executive at the "top level of the power structure" and as a "corporate officer" documents this trend toward expanded strategic management responsibilities.[5]

Some nursing administrators are more involved in strategic decisions than others due to their position in the organizational hierarchy. For example, the American Nurses' Association, in its statement of "Roles, Responsibilities, and Qualifications for Nurse Administrators,"[6] identifies three levels of nursing administrative practice: the first line level, the middle level, and the executive level. The primary responsibility of the first line nurse administrator is the "direction of staff members in the delivery of nursing care." At the middle level, the nurse administrator provides a link between first line administration and executive management. A key part of this role is to "provide clinical and administrative expertise to the units' first line administrators."

At the executive level, the nurse administrator (or nurse executive) is "responsible for the nursing department and manages from the perspective of the organization as a whole." The planning perspective is long (five to ten years), with a significant part of the role involving participation in top management decision making, including the establishment of financial and organizational goals.

More recently the American Hospital Association's Council on Nursing and the American Organization of Nurse Executives jointly developed a statement describing the role and functions of the hospital nurse executive. According to this statement, the nurse executive participates in financial forecasting and planning, along with other members of the executive management team. The nurse executive has the responsibility to articulate nursing's contributions to the financial viability of the institution, and the resources necessary for patient care. It is the responsibility of the nurse executive to establish and maintain a financial plan for nursing that integrates the institution's missions and goals.[7]

Financial management skills are clearly an important prerequisite for effective completion of the nursing administrator's job responsibilities.

The final report of the Institute of Medicine's study *Nursing and Nursing Education: Public Policies and Private Actions* specifically states that there was "widespread conviction among administrators of hospitals and long-term care facilities that their nurse administrator colleagues could make the delivery of the care more cost effective if they had better grounding in financial management" and that "nurse administrators should be able to contribute to executive management decisions beyond nursing services."[8] The nursing administrators' familiarity with all aspects of hospital operations gives them the unique opportunity to contribute to a better understanding of cost-sensitive issues as well as to participate in executive level decision making to develop institution-wide cost containment programs.

In this book we provide an overview of the financial management function for nursing administrators. The discussion assumes no formal training in accounting or finance, but it does assume exposure to the financial management requirements in the acute care setting. It is directed primarily to executive level nursing administrators who wish to participate more actively in institutional financial management.

The book differs from finance texts in health or hospital administration in its emphasis on a nursing perspective. In addition, it differs from more traditional nursing administration texts in its concentration on financial management of the institution, but once again from the nursing perspective.

In establishing a context for understanding the importance of financial management activities, this chapter explores some of the recent trends that are exerting an impact on hospital financial management. These pressures are escalating the financial management function to the forefront in hospital administration. We believe that the nursing administrator is in a unique position and that this position carries with it certain major responsibilities. These responsibilities center primarily on the ability to integrate financial demands and pressures that may erode the quality of clinical care.

AN OVERVIEW OF HEALTH CARE COSTS

The passage of Medicare and Medicaid during the Johnson administration ushered in a period of national health policy with the aim of promoting access to health care for those who had previously been disenfranchised from it—the poor and the elderly. This policy was implemented through federal initiatives that expanded both the number of providers and the number of facilities. It also established a reimbursement system to support this expansion. As Table 1–1 indicates, health care spending increased from slightly less than $27 billion in 1960 to over $387 billion in 1984. This increase represents a doubling in the proportion of gross national product spent on health care.

A review of the literature[9] indicates that there have in fact been significant changes in the health status of the American people in the past 20 years. For example, during the period from 1968 to 1980 there was an overall 20 percent reduction in death rates, with a 72 percent decrease in the death rate from childbirth, a 53 percent decrease in deaths due to pneumonia and influenza, a 52 percent decrease in deaths from tuberculosis, and a 31 percent decrease in deaths from diabetes.[10] The health policy of increased access can also be viewed as successful because, according to the Congressional Budget Office report in 1983, 95 percent of elderly persons had hospital coverage under Medicare.[11]

The development of new drugs, noninvasive diagnostic procedures, and decreased incidence of rejection reactions following transplant surgery made possible by the introduction of cyclosporine has led to an increase in the number of lives that may be improved or saved. It has also raised ethical issues with regard to the appropriate criteria for patient selection for transplantation.

More recently, however, with budget deficits growing at an alarming rate, federal and state policy makers have begun to realize that the nation's financial resources are not unlimited. Part of that realization has resulted in an intensive examination of the rapidly rising costs of health care. Consequently, federal policy

Table 1–1 National Health Expenditures and Percent of GNP for Selected Years 1960–1984

Calendar Year	GNP (Billions)	National Health Expenditures Amount (Billions)	Per capita	Percent of GNP
1960	$ 506.5	$ 26.9	$ 146	5.3
1965	691.0	41.7	211	6.0
1970	992.7	74.7	358	7.5
1975	1,549.2	132.7	590	8.6
1980	2,631.7	248.0	1,049	9.4
1981	2,957.8	285.8	1,197	9.7
1983	3,304.8	355.1	1,461	10.7
1984	3,662.8	387.4	1,580	10.6

Sources: Health Care Financing Review, Vol. 5, No. 3, p. 7, Spring 1984, and *HHS News*, July 31, 1985, press release, U.S. Department of Health and Human Services.

has been reoriented to the goal of constraining the increase in health care costs. The development of business coalitions and the active involvement of private enterprise have given added impetus to federal efforts to control costs.

Corporate spending on health care doubled from 1960 to 1980, to $90 billion a year. This represented almost four percent of corporate GNP.[12] Business spending on health care in 1984 was almost equal to after-tax corporate profits. The response by some corporate businesses has been to provide plans for employees encouraging them to join capitated health plans. In fact, Iglehart suggests that the

> single most compelling force [behind the movement toward HMOs] is the mounting perception among large public and private purchasers that fee-for-service medicine, left unfettered by limitations on the patient's choice of physician and by other mechanisms intended to promote cost consciousness, simply lacks the discipline necessary to reduce the volume of services delivered, particularly inpatient care, and thereby check the growth of expenditures.[13]

As corporations pressure health organizations for greater cost control, it is likely that the number of prepaid plans will expand.

THE CHANGING NATURE OF COMPETITION IN THE HEALTH INDUSTRY

Prior to the implementation of prospective payment legislation, competition among hospitals primarily took place in the area of services offered and physician recruitment. There was no price competition, nor was there a need for hospitals to manage their human, material, or financial resources efficiently. Hospitals, in general, attempted to make themselves more attractive to patients and physicians by having more and better staff, and by having a larger and more luxurious or more comfortable physical plant, all of which enabled the hospital to treat a wider variety of patients and provide a higher level of service.[14]

Competition, as an economic concept, is based on a number of assumptions, many of which may not apply to the health care industry. It is important to understand these assumptions, why there is debate about their relevance to health care, and how these are changing in the light of reimbursement reform. Figure 1–1 represents some of the relationships that have an impact on competition in health care. Each factor in the figure is discussed in detail below.

The first area in which hospital competition differs from competition in other industries is the pervasiveness of third party coverage for health services. The effect is to remove the link between consumer sensitivity to and payment of services because actual out-of-pocket expenses are minimal. Contributing to this

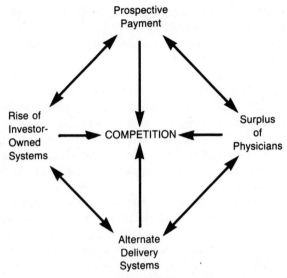

Figure 1–1 The Changing Nature of Competition in Health Care

is the general expectation among providers (as well as recipients of care) that individuals would seek the highest possible quality of care, regardless of price, and regardless of whether or not the extent and intensity of care were in fact necessary. In other words, patients were able to receive, and institutions were able to provide, as much high quality care as possible, whether or not the actual additional expenditures for that care led to any measurable improvement in patient outcomes.

A second way in which competition in health care deviates from the classical model is that most hospitals are not-for-profit entities, while theories of competition are based on the assumption that firms wish to maximize profits. This profit orientation of the competitive model leads to an internal focus on costs and prices as the basis for economic decision making within the firm. Therefore, decisions about which products will be produced, and in what volume, are made on the basis of the extent to which that product contributes to net profit for the firm. If a product is, for any reason, not successful from an economic point of view, the product is discontinued. Hospitals, at least nonprofit hospitals, have not had this bottom-line orientation until recently. Therefore, decisions about services tended more often than not to be made on the basis of noneconomic and occasionally nonrational criteria. They were frequently based on the subjective judgments of powerful individuals on the medical staff or governing board.

The third deviation from traditional economic theory is the role that physicians play in creating a market for health services. The issue of ''physician-induced demand'' for health services is a controversial one that has not been exhaustively researched. Irrespective of the inability to firmly lay the issue to rest, there is no question that physicians serve as intermediaries between consumers of health care and institutional providers of health care. In this role, physicians serve their own economic and professional interests. In the past, there was little reason for this not to occur. The lay public believed that only physicians could make decisions about whether or not health services were required, and that only physicians could make judgments about the extensiveness of those services. Consumers were willing to abdicate their responsibility for determining the need for health services. The "medicalization" of social problems (e.g., alcoholism, drug addiction, and similar problems) further expanded the power of physicians to control consumer decisions about health services.[14]

Several developments within the last five years markedly changed the nature of competition in the health care industry. These changes, while often discussed independently, must be viewed as interdependent. Taken altogether, they have dramatically, and perhaps forever, altered the course of institutional health care delivery in this country.

The one event that has had the most dramatic impact on health care delivery was the passage in 1983 of Medicare prospective pricing legislation (PPS). Briefly, PPS pays hospitals preestablished prices for each of 467 diagnosis related groups. If the hospital is able to treat the patient for less than the price for the DRG, the hospital may retain the reimbursed amount. If, however, the hospital overspends on a patient's hospital stay, it must make up the difference.

DRG stands for Diagnosis Related Group. DRGs are basically case mix indicators. Although there are many uses for developing valid case mix indices, such as research and policy decisions, we are primarily interested in case mix indices and utilization (and therefore costs) of hospital resources. For this purpose, a case mix measure should help predict discrete patterns of utilization that account for cost differences. DRGs are simply a classification scheme for predicting what kind of patients (diagnoses) will use what kind of services and how much these services will cost.

DRGs were developed in the late 1960s as an outgrowth of utilization review. To determine if a patient's length of stay was appropriate, some kind of standard had to be uniformly applied. The original research on development of DRGs was done at Yale University. Starting with 83 major diagnostic categories (MDCs), and with a computer program called AutoGrp, diagnoses were classified so they were homogeneous with respect to length of stay, as well as being similar medically. Three hundred eighty-three of these "diagnosis related groups" were originally identified. In a second iteration of the process, increased emphasis was placed on clinical information and organ systems rather than on etiology and statistics. Twenty-three MDCs were identified, from which 476 DRGs were developed. The splits used in this round, which make up the DRG system under which hospitals are now operating, were presence of surgical procedure, presence of complication or comorbid condition, and age.

Prior to the implementation of DRGs, reimbursement for hospitals was based on costs and was determined after treatment had been rendered. In other words, and in oversimplified terms, whatever it cost the hospital to provide care, cost-based retrospective reimbursement covered it. Because hospitals knew that they would recover essentially whatever they spent, the incentives were to do more lab tests, more procedures, more x-rays. There were absolutely no incentives to operate efficiently.

In 1982, TEFRA (the Tax Equity and Fiscal Responsibility Act) mandated that hospitals should be paid, for treatment of Medicare patients, on a cost per *patient stay* basis, and that ceilings and caps would be placed on reimbursement. TEFRA was the first legislative action directed specifically at radical reform in the approach to reimbursement. Then, on April 20, 1983, PL 98-21, the Social Security Amendment of 1983, was signed into law, mandating that prices (rather than costs) be fixed at the beginning of the hospital's fiscal year. Prospective payment was to be phased in over a three-year period. During the first year, payment for each DRG was to be based on 75 percent of the hospital-specific cost per case plus 25 percent of the regional average price for the DRG. In year two, the proportion would move to 50 percent of the hospital-specific cost per case amount plus 37.5 percent of the regional average price for the patient's DRG plus 12.5 percent of the national average price. In year three, the proportions would change to 25 percent of the hospital-specific cost per case plus 37.5 percent of the regional average price for the DRG plus 37.5 percent of the national average price. Finally, in the fourth year, payments were to have been based on the urban or rural national average price for each DRG, adjusted for differences in geographic area wage rates.

In addition, each hospital's cost per case limit was to be adjusted using a hospital-specific case mix index based on the complexity of treatment patients received as a group in that hospital. This case mix index was developed using the Medicare Provider Analysis and Review (MEDPAR) files as well as data from Medicare cost reports. For example, a case mix index of 1.0 indicates that the hospital delivers care of "average" complexity, while a case mix index greater than 1.0 indicates that, on the whole, care is more complex than "average." Similarly, a case mix index of less than 1.0 indicates that, on the whole, patients require somewhat less than average complexity of care. The designated cost per case, also determined through MEDPAR files and Medicare cost reports, is then multiplied by the case mix index in order to adjust reimbursement levels for complexity of care. For example, academic medical centers, with their high costs of medical education and technology, will tend to have higher case mix indices than community hospitals.

Prospective payment covers, at present, only inpatient services. For the first three years of prospective payment, capital expenses (depreciation, interest, and lease expense, return on equity for investor-owned hospitals) were reimbursed on a cost basis as a "pass-through." Similarly, direct and indirect costs of approved medical education programs were also treated as a pass-through cost. Currently, future treatment of capital and educational expenses is being debated. The issues underlying the debate, however, are beyond the scope of this book.

The critical point for the nurse administrator is that prospective payment changed even the nonprofit hospital into an institution driven by finances. Without a full understanding of these changes, the nursing administrator loses a significant degree of control and therefore also diminishes effectiveness.

Competition between hospitals has tended to be nonprice competition. Resources are no longer available for hospitals to expand staff, services, and physical plant. Hospitals now must develop management systems to identify costs of various services and programs and develop management strategies to control these costs. As occupancy rates and lengths of stay continue to decrease, hospitals will have even less patient services revenue available and will need to look at ways of expanding nonpatient services, as well as other diversification strategies.

As business and industry have responded aggressively to the billions of dollars in costs for employee health coverage, they are having an enormous impact on how employees seek health services. In the past it was typical for large corporations to provide first dollar coverage for employees and their families. This led to increased levels of demand. However, congressional testimony in 1983 found that, in a survey of 1,400 companies, in the two years between 1980 and 1982, 34 percent had increased copayments for inpatient hospital care.

In other companies, employees are provided the choice of enrolling in a variety of health maintenance organizations or preferred provider organizations, and in still other companies, employees *must* enroll in some type of capitated health plan. The net effect of the increase in payment of out-of-pocket expenses is that consumers of health care services are becoming more sensitive to health care costs.

Another significant change is that consumers are no longer totally dependent upon physicians for decisions about health services. For example, the increase in nonphysician providers like nurse practitioners, and the general change in social awareness of health, have given consumers additional knowledge that they now are using. They are making decisions about health care, rather than relying on physicians. The dramatic increase in smoking cessation programs, programs for weight reduction, the focus on health and fitness, and related factors has changed the health status of some individuals. For many it has changed their outlook about health, so that they are less likely to seek health services for perceived problems.

The presence and activity of the investor-owned hospital chains have also had a remarkable effect on competition in health care. These hospitals brought to the industry a marketing orientation that is beginning to pervade the nonprofit sector. Prior to prospective pricing legislation, the approach of the investor-owned hospital systems was viewed quite negatively. Arnold Relman, perhaps the most widely known critic of the for-profit sector, dubbed it the "new medical-industrial complex."[15] Yet the strategies utilized by the for-profit sector are now being adopted to some extent by the nonprofit sector as it attempts to adapt to the bottom-line orientation demanded by prospective payment. Despite the enormous success of the investor-owned hospitals during the later 1970s and early 1980s, as of early 1986 occupancy rates in investor-owned hospital chains were approximately 50–60 percent, while occupancy rates in nonprofit community hospitals were in the range of 65–70 percent.

THE RISE OF MULTI-INSTITUTIONAL ARRANGEMENTS

Growth of the investor-owned hospital industry began in the late 1960s when the passage of Medicare and Medicaid created large demand for government-paid health services. Fledgling investor-owned hospitals, however, often found themselves undercapitalized, unable to control inflationary expenses, and incapable of dealing with increasingly complex government regulations.[16] Hospital management companies developed in response to the need for expertise in finance and administration. Since 1978, the number of beds in investor-owned systems has increased 20.7 percent; the number of hospitals in investor-owned systems has increased 23.1 percent. Net revenues for the five largest hospital management companies—Hospital Corporation of American (HCA), Humana, American Medical International (AMI), National Medical Enterprises (NME), and Life-mark—nearly tripled, from $1.8 billion in 1976 to $5.48 billion in 1981. Yet, despite this rapid growth, investor-owned hospital systems operate only 11 percent of this country's hospital beds.[17]

Differences between Hospital Types

To understand the impact of the growth of the investor-owned hospital systems, it is important to compare how they differ legally, financially, and organizationally from nonprofit hospitals.

Legal Differences

Nonprofit hospitals are most often operated as not-for-profit corporations and are governed by state corporation laws. These statutes generally require that the corporation be formed for a charitable, educational, or scientific purpose.[18] The income and assets of the nonprofit corporation are not permitted to benefit any private individual directly. In contrast, investor-owned hospitals are operated either as separate proprietary businesses or as subsidiaries of larger profit-making multihospital systems. Investor-owned hospitals are also governed by the business corporation laws of the states in which they are incorporated.

Because of the general lack of restrictions on the kinds of businesses that can be conducted by a corporation, investor-owned hospitals are free to diversify into related as well as unrelated businesses.[19] While nonprofit hospitals may also enter other businesses, to do so may require restructuring of the nonprofit corporation, as well as careful review of whether or not the new business will qualify for tax-exempt status.

Financial Differences

The primary factor differentiating nonprofit from investor-owned hospitals is exemption from federal income tax under Section 501(c)(3) of the Internal Revenue Code. Tax-exempt status is also important because it provides access to other sources of support, such as tax-deductible philanthropic donations and tax-exempt bonds. Other savings that accrue to the nonprofit hospital include exemptions from state property tax, state sales tax, and corporate income tax.

While nonprofit hospitals may have an advantage as a result of tax treatment, investor-owned hospitals have access to a source of capital denied to nonprofit hospitals: raising equity through issuing stock. Freestanding nonprofit hospitals are further disadvantaged because certain financial instruments such as revenue bonds require a strong financial base to achieve investment grade ratings, something individual nonprofit hospitals may have difficulty attaining. It should be noted, however, that independent investor-owned hospitals may also have difficulty achieving a strong financial position.

The investor-owned hospital industry has one of the highest levels of borrowing in this country, with debt ranging from 60 to 85 percent of capital structure. Because of the stability and predictability of their profits, as well as guaranteed revenue under charge-based reimbursement, the investor-owned hospitals have been able to convince the financial and investment communities that they are able to support such debt levels.[20,21] Investor-owned hospitals are therefore able to obtain funds quickly, under favorable conditions, thereby allowing them to move rapidly when opportunities arise. Nonprofit hospitals, on the other hand, generally borrow for specific projects and may experience delays in funding due to thorough evaluation of their debt capacity.

Another factor differentiating investor-owned from nonprofit hospitals is related to reimbursement factors. Many nonprofit hospitals have been faced with having to make up shortfalls in Medicare reimbursement by shifting costs to paying patients or commercial insurance carriers. In contrast, investor-owned hospitals may choose not to participate in Medicare and some may deny treatment to indigent patients. This choice may not be available to nonprofit hospitals whose social mission involves treatment of patients regardless of ability to pay. In addition, nonprofit hospitals may be obligated to provide indigent care as a condition of having received Hill-Burton funds.

Organizational Differences

Investor-owned and nonprofit hospitals vary in the way in which they adapt to requirements relating to provision of patient care, as well as to demands of the increasingly complex environments in which they operate. The differences emerge, in part, due to constraints imposed by their legal and financial characteristics. The dissimilarities are accentuated in the strategies they employ to achieve their missions and goals. This is best explained by briefly examining the evolution of the hospital as a community institution.

Community hospitals originally received financial support through philanthropic contributions from wealthy members of the community. In return these individuals frequently were awarded a seat on the hospital's board of trustees. The arrangement suited all those involved: physicians had a place to treat their patients and they increased their legitimacy in the community by their association with prominent citizens. Sponsors, in serving community interests, also served their own.[22]

Over time, the typical community hospital evolved into an institution attempting to be responsive to multiple constituent groups. Yet the hospital had no formal mechanism to reconcile or even provide an arena for discussion of the frequently conflicting demands of these groups. Until recently, there had been no impetus to do so.

The original proprietary hospitals tended to be located in small towns and cities of the West. They were small, not very elaborate, and tended to serve paying patients almost entirely.[23] While these original proprietary hospitals disappeared during the 1940s, at least one critical aspect of their organization remained: their emphasis on serving the needs of physicians. In today's investor-owned hospitals, boards are frequently dominated by insiders and physicians, narrowing the range of interests that must be addressed.

Larson suggests that, when combined with the presence of a sophisticated strategic planning process, this goal congruence allows consensus to develop and action to be taken quickly on key moves.[24] Investor-owned hospitals have often capitalized on opportunities to expand and serve new markets, or conversely, to abandon services in markets that were not profitable. This marketing obligation challenges long and dearly held assumptions about the obligation of hospitals to provide care to anyone in need, regardless of ability to pay, and has been one of the main points of contention cited by critics of the organized for-profit industry.

In a review of the literature on multihospital systems, Ermann and Gabel outlined the touted advantages of multihospital systems compared with independent freestanding hospitals.[25] These benefits were grouped in three categories: economic benefits; personnel and management benefits; and planning, program, and organization benefits.

Economic benefits for multihospital systems include access to the capital necessary for replacement, renovation, or expansion. Favorable borrowing terms are available to multihospital systems due to lenders' perception of lower risk because of multihospital systems' stronger financial position. Such favorable conditions provide for lower levels of debt service that must be covered from operating revenues, thereby decreasing some pressures on sources of operating revenues.

A second benefit is the economies of scale available through volume purchasing arrangements. Systems may be able to share costly high technology services and equipment, thereby creating additional levels of efficiency and productivity. A third economic benefit is the ability to diversify. As sources of patient-service revenue become more constrained under prospective payment legislation, it has become critical for hospitals to enter other lines of business.

Personnel management benefits refer to the ability of systems to attract and retain high-level clinical and management personnel, and to provide ample opportunities for mobility, both laterally and promotionally, within the system. However, individuals within systems may also experience corporate bureaucratic interference and a lack of autonomy. Planning benefits include the ability to better assess regional and state needs, as well as the ability to effectively influence local and regional planning agencies.

Ermann and Gabel point out, however, that while the empirical literature *does* support the favored position of multihospital systems in capital markets, all other conclusions are still tentative. Therefore, the advantages of multihospital systems may not be any more substantial than those of freestanding institutions.

ALTERNATIVE DELIVERY SYSTEMS

The rapid growth of alternative delivery systems, broadly defined to include new ways of providing care within the acute care setting, has also contributed to the changing nature of competition in health care. Health maintenance organizations (HMOs), preferred provider organizations (PPOs), ambulatory care centers, surgicenters, and satellite clinics are all examples of these new types of arrangements. We will focus primarily on HMOs and PPOs, their description, growth, and future. This will relate closely to the final topic of this chapter—the changing nature of physician-hospital relationships.

Health Maintenance Organizations

Health maintenance organizations had their beginnings in 1933 when Dr. Sidney Garfield offered to provide health care to ill workmen if insurers prepaid him five cents a day. That was the beginning of the Kaiser prepaid health plan that, following World War II, was extended to citizens of the community.

The federal government enacted the Health Maintenance Organization Act in 1973, as part of the attempt by the Nixon administration to introduce competition into the health care environment. In the decade from 1973 to 1983, the federal government provided $364 million in grants and loans for the development of HMOs. In 1984, enrollment in prepaid health plans was over 17 million.[26]

An HMO has been defined as:

> any organization, profit or non-profit, that accepts responsibility for the provision and delivery of a predetermined set of comprehensive health maintenance and treatment services to a voluntarily enrolled group for a negotiated and fixed periodic capitation payment.[27]

The key aspects of this definition need to be reviewed.

First, the HMO undertakes a contractual responsibility to provide an identified set of health services. Second, the HMO has a defined, enrolled population that allows it, in contrast with the traditional fee-for-service arrangement, to more accurately forecast demand for services. Third, the population enrolled in an HMO is enrolled voluntarily and on an individual basis and has the option of expressing dissatisfaction with services by choosing to disenroll. Fourth, the HMO is paid a fixed amount (i.e., on a capitation basis) at periodic intervals, and this payment is independent of services rendered to enrollees. Finally, the HMO is "at risk" financially. In other words, if more care is given than was paid for, the HMO itself sustains the financial loss.[28]

Although there are variations in the structure and organization of health maintenance organizations, there are essentially three basic types. One type is the prepaid group practice, where physicians are paid on a salary or capitation basis. The second type, the independent practice association (IPA), works on the basis of independent community physicians billing the HMO directly for services provided to HMO enrollees. The third type, the network HMO, involves contracts between two or more group practices to provide health services.

The difference between the traditional fee-for-service arrangement and the health maintenance organization concept is that HMOs combine the functions of health insurance and health care delivery in the same organization. The staff model is the most integrated type of HMO; employees of the HMO deliver care and are therefore at risk for excess utilization of HMO services. In a group model HMO there are two organizations, of which the HMO is at risk. Physicians and other clinical and nonclinical employees are employed by the group, or are partners in the group. The HMO itself has a contract with the group to provide services. In an independent practice association (IPA) model, physicians are generally in private practice in the community. The HMO can contract with, and remain at risk for, physicians who typically receive payment on a fee-for-service basis. The advantage to members of an IPA is that there remains some freedom of choice with regard to the physician they will be seeing.

Luft, after reviewing the performance of HMOs, finds that in all cases the total cost of medical care for HMO enrollees is lower than for comparable people with conventional insurance coverage.[29] In prepaid group practices, total costs range from 10 to 40 percent below fee-for-service payments. Yet he also concludes that these decreased costs result primarily from lower hospital utilization and suggests that lower costs do not result from "substantially lower costs per unit of service."

More recent studies similarly find that hospitalization rates are significantly lower for HMO enrollees.[30,31] These studies also found that the lower hospitalization rate is not due to the practice of selecting enrollees who are least likely to need health services. Rather, lower hospitalization rates, and therefore lower costs, are achieved through advanced screening when hospitalization appears to be necessary, increased utilization of outpatient services, careful monitoring of length of stay, and provision of home health care services when necessary.

The second type of organized alternative delivery system, the preferred provider organization, has the following characteristics:[32]

- a provider panel with a limited number of physicians and hospitals
- a negotiated fee schedule, which most often contains some sort of discount
- consumers who are not "locked in" but have additional benefits associated with use of PPO providers
- quick turnaround on provider claims

Despite the diversity in sponsorship of preferred provider organizations, their structure is basically quite simple. It consists of a panel of providers—hospital and physicians—in some combination. The only agreement that locks the provider and the consumer together is that "each time a designated service is provided by this panel, it is provided at a previously agreed upon fee. There is no prepayment or capitation amount paid to the providers, unlike health maintenance organizations."[33] Consumers are not locked in, but they are offered financial rewards, such as waiver of copayments and deductibles or improved benefits, to use a provider associated with the preferred group.

The negotiated (i.e., discounted) price is acceptable to hospital and physician providers for several reasons. First is the rapid turnaround on claims payment that enhances the organization's cash flow. The second is that despite the discounted fees, association with the preferred provider organization tends to increase the providers' volume of patients and therefore of services delivered.

The American Hospital Association first identified 33 PPOs in 1982, and by 1984 the American Association of Preferred Provider Organizations reported 143 PPOs operating. A number of factors support the growth of PPOs.[34] The first factor is clearly the interest and concern of major purchasers of health care coverage—employers. An outcome of employer interest has been the development of employer-dominated health care coalitions formed specifically to address the issue of increasing health care costs.[35] However, whether or not PPOs are effective in decreasing health care costs is yet to be determined.

Other arrangements are also having an impact by changing the way health care is delivered. These include primary care management programs, delivery of more intensive levels of care in outpatient settings, preadmission testing, ambulatory surgery, same-day surgery, freestanding emergency centers, and so forth. While no one is willing to make predictions about the specific effects of these arrangements, there is consensus that they are having an impact.

EFFECTS OF THE EXCESS OF PHYSICIANS

Since physicians play a major role in determining the level of health care expenditures, it is important to examine how the projected surplus of physicians will have an impact on competition in health care. First, we will briefly describe how the physician surplus evolved.

The number of physicians grew from 220,000 in 1950 to over 500,000 in 1982.[36] Two federal programs provided the impetus for this expansion. The first, which began following World War II, was federal financing of medical schools through research grants. The enactment in 1963 of the Health Professions Educational Assistance Act, the amendments passed in 1971 as part of the Comprehensive Health Manpower Training Act, as well as the Health Professions Educational Assistance Act of 1976, led to a dramatic increase in the number of medical schools. In 1961, there were 68 medical schools in the United States; by 1983, there were 127.[37]

The second major contributor to the growth in the supply of physicians was the influx of foreign-trained medical graduates (FMGs). The Department of Health and Human Services reports that in the ten years from 1970 to 1980 the number of physicians trained in the United States increased by about one-third, while the number of FMGs increased by more than two-thirds.[38] In an effort to decrease the supply of FMGs in this country, as part of the Health Professions Educational Assistance Act of 1976, immigration restrictions were placed on aliens. In addition, a more difficult medical examination was required.

Two reports have specifically addressed the issue of physician supply: the Graduate Medical Education National Advisory Committee (GMENAC)[39] in 1980, and the Department of Health and Human Services in 1984.[40] Both estimate a future excess aggregate supply of physicians. The GMENAC report predicted an excess of 70,000 physicians by 1990 and 145,000 by 2000. HHS predicted an excess of 25,000 by 1990 and 52,000 by the year 2000. This increase represents growth three times faster than in the past 20 years, when the growth of the American economy was considerably greater than what most experts predict it will be in the 1980s and 1990s.[41] Another factor clearly differentiating the 1960s and 1970s from the 1980s and 1990s is that the national health policy of the past 20 years has been to increase access and expand the availability of health care services, while today and in the future, policy is to constrain costs if not limit access.

According to the GAO's review of the literature, there are differences of opinion regarding whether an excess of physicians will result in an increase or a decrease in health expenditures.[42] Those who believe that an oversupply of physicians will result in increased health expenditures cite three reasons for their view. First, in a market characterized by permanent excess demand, more physicians may simply reduce the percentage of unmet demand. Second, much of the demand for other health care services (i.e., not just physician services but hospital care and drugs) is generated by physicians. And third, physicians may seek to maintain a target level of individual income, despite decreased demand for their services, simply by increasing professional fees.

Those who suggest that the excess of physicians will decrease expenditures for health care cite the competition between physicians for patients, and between hospitals and physicians to serve as the primary source of patient treatment. Many more physicians are choosing to join alternative delivery systems and receive a salary because of the increased competition in private practice, the excessive level of debt that the young medical graduate carries, the expenses of setting up and maintaining a profitable private practice, and the cost of malpractice insurance.

The increased supply of physicians is likely to have a significant impact on the relationships that physicians have with hospitals. Combined with the imperatives of prospective payment that demand much closer scrutiny of physician practice patterns in the hospital setting, rough roads may lie ahead for physicians. The oversupply of physicians may, however, bode well for those individuals who hold appointments on staffs of prestigious hospitals, since admitting privileges are likely to be cut in an effort to maintain a smaller staff size. In addition, physicians will work diligently to protect their volume of work and, no less importantly, their income.

The increase in the number of physicians is also likely to lead to decreasing income, or at least incomes that rise at a less steady rate. Combined with increasing administrative control over physician practice patterns in the hospital setting, lower incomes may alter the work patterns of physicians. Some may seek additional employment, others may institute more flexible hours, seeing patients during the evening or on Saturdays. House calls may also return. All of this will increase the number of physicians who are willing to practice in group settings where there is less demand to be on call, a wide range of professional colleagueship, and less financial drain to establish a private practice.

A recent article in *American Medical News*[44] said,

For the first time in decades, a buyer's market is developing in medicine. As more open slots appear in appointment books and incomes show signs of slipping, many physicians are sensing seismic tremors beneath the once stable medical terrain. . . . Not many physicians are doing acrobatics yet, but many are making drastic changes in their practices, substituting new practice arrangements for old ones, and behaving increasingly like businessmen.

FINANCIAL MANAGEMENT RESPONSIBILITIES IN A CHANGING CONTEXT

What are the financial management responsibilities of nurse administrators considering the changing context of health care costs, competition, multi-institutional arrangements, alternative delivery systems, and an excess supply of physicians? This is the question to which the remainder of this book is devoted. However, it is appropriate to underscore the fact that unless nursing administrators understand the changing context described above, and are willing to try to define the implications for their nursing unit, program, department, or organization, then substantial expertise in financial management concepts will be relatively meaningless. Nurse administrators' financial responsibilities are dependent on and shaped by the ever-changing context of the health care field.

As we have seen, the shift from a cost-based reimbursement system to a method of prospective price determination has dramatically introduced incentives for hospitals to attempt to operate efficiently. Nursing administrators are increasingly called upon to institute financial controls for attaining efficiency. In addition, the growth of multi-institutional systems has lead to an examination of some of the assumptions on which hospital care has been based. Nursing administrators are taking an active role in determining the trade-offs between quality of care and financial performance. The proliferation of alternative delivery systems, in addition, has had an impact on competition, as has the projected surplus of physicians.

Ultimately these factors have forced health care organizations and nursing administrators to become attuned to "bottom-line" financial performance if they expect to survive the next five years. Nursing administrators have a unique contribution to make in this evolution, but they will be effective on the top management team only if they increase their understanding of financial management concepts.

NOTES

1. American Hospital Association, *Role, Functions and Qualifications of the Nursing Service Administrator in a Health Care Institution* (Chicago: AHA, 1979).

2. National Commission on Nursing, *Initial Report and Preliminary Recommendations* (Chicago: AHA, 1981).

3. R. Shirley, "Limiting the Scope of Strategy: A Decision-based Approach," *Academy of Management Review* 7, no. 2 (1982): 262–268.

4. C. Weisman, C. Alexander, and L. Morlock, "Hospital Decision-making: What Is Nursing's Role?" *Journal of Nursing Administration* 11 (1981): 31–36.

5. Muriel Poulin, "The Nurse Executive Role: A Structural and Functional Analysis," *Journal of Nursing Administration*, no. 14 (February 1984): 9–14.

6. American Nurses' Association, *Roles, Responsibilities, and Qualifications for Nurse Administrators* (Chicago: AHA, 1978).

7. American Hospital Association, *Role and Function of the Hospital Nurse Executive* (Chicago: AHA, 1985).

8. Institute of Medicine, *Nursing and Nursing Education: Public Policies and Private Action* (Washington, D.C.: National Academy Press, 1981).

9. U.S. General Accounting Office, *How Health Maintenance Organizations Control Costs* (Washington, D.C.: GAO, HRD-82-31, December 29, 1981).

10. D. Rogers et al, "Who Needs Medicaid?" *New England Journal of Medicine* 307, no. 1 (July 1, 1982):16.

11. U.S. Congressional Budget Office, *Changing the Structure of Medicare Benefits: Issues and Options* (Washington, D.C.: CBO, March 1983).

12. Fern Chapman, "Deciding Who Pays to Save Lives," *Fortune*, May 27, 1985, pp. 59–70.

13. John K. Iglehart, "HMOs (For Profit and Not For Profit) on the Move," *New England Journal of Medicine* 310, no. 18 (1984): 1203–1208.

14. Renee Fox, "The Medicalization and Demedicalization of American Society," in John Knowles, ed., *Doing Better and Feeling Worse* (New York: W.W. Norton & Company, 1977).

15. Arnold Relman, "The New Medical Industrial Complex," *New England Journal of Medicine* 309, no. 6 (1981): 370–372.

16. A. Roth, "Note on the Hospital Management Industry," Case No. 9-377-169 (Cambridge: Harvard Business School, 1976).

17. Federation of American Hospitals, *Directory of Investor-owned Hospitals and Hospital Management Companies* (Little Rock, Ark: Federation of American Hospitals, 1982).

18. J. Horty and D. Mulholland, "Legal Differences between Investor-owned and Non-profit Health Care Institutions," in B. Gray, ed., *The New Health Care for Profit* (Washington, D.C.: National Academy Press, 1983).

19. Ibid.

20. C. Sherman and J. Thompson, *Hospital Management: Industry Update* (New York: Prudential-Bache Securities, 1983).

21. R. Siegrist, "Wall Street and the For-profit Hospital Management Companies," in B. Gray, ed., *The New Health Care for Profit* (Washington, D.C.: National Academy Press, 1983).

22. Paul Starr, *The Social Transformation of American Medicine* (New York: Basic Books, 1982).

23. Ibid.

24. J. Larson, "Factors in the Success of the Investor-owned Hospitals: Implications for the Not-for-profits," *Hospital and Health Service Administration* 28 (1983): 43–49.

25. D. Ermann and J. Gabel, "Multihospital Systems: Issues and Empirical Findings," *Health Affairs* 3, no. 1 (1984): 50–64.

26. InterStudy, 1984 National HMO Census (Excelsior, Minn.: Interstudy).

27. R. Shouldice and K. Shouldice, *Medical Group Practice and Health Maintenance Organizations* (Washington, D.C.: Information Resources Press, 1978).

28. Harold Luft, "Assessing the Evidence on HMO Performance," *Milbank Memorial Fund Quarterly* 58, no. 4 (1980): 501–536.

29. Ibid.

30. W. Manning et al., "A Controlled Trial of the Effect of a Prepaid Group Practice on the Use of Services," *New England Journal of Medicine* 310, no. 23 (June 7, 1984): 1505.

31. Iglehart, "HMOs."

32. Linda Ellwein and David Gregg, "InterStudy Researchers Trace Progress of PPOs, Provide Insight into Future Growth," *FAH Review* (July-August 1982): 20–25.

33. Ibid.

34. Jon Gabel and D. Ermann, "Preferred Provider Organizations: Performance, Problems, and Promise," *Health Affairs* 4, no. 1 (Spring 1985): 24–40.

35. Mark Reisler, "Business in Richmond Attacks Health Care Costs," *Harvard Business Review* 63, no. 1 (January-February 1985): 145–155.

36. American Medical Association, *The American Health Care System* (Chicago, Ill.: AMA, 1984).

37. U.S. Department of Health and Human Services, *Summary Report of the Graduate Medical Education National Advisory Committee to the Secretary* (Washington, D.C.: DHHS, September 1980).

38. U.S. Department of Health and Human Services, *Third Report to the President and Congress on the Status of Health Professions Personnel* (Washington, D.C.: DHHS, January 1982).

39. Carol Golin, "Competition Forces Changes in Practices," *American Medical News*, January 3, 1986, p. 28.

40. U.S. Department of Health and Human Services, *Report to the President and Congress on the Status of Health Professions Personnel* (Washington, D.C.: DHHS, May 1984).

41. Eli Ginzberg, et al., "The Expanding Physician Supply and Health Policy: The Crowded Outlook," *Milbank Memorial Fund Quarterly* 59, no. 4 (Fall 1981): 508–541.

42. U.S. Government Accounting Office, *Constraining National Health Care Expenditures: Achieving Quality Care at an Affordable Cost* (Washington, D.C.: GAO, September 30, 1985).

43. Ginzberg et al., "Expanding Physician Supply."

44. Golin, "Competition."

Chapter 2

Financial Concepts, Statements, and Reports

Nursing administrators responsible for managing the financial performance of a work unit, department, program, division, or organization must be capable of communicating effectively with other managers. This responsibility demands a capacity for speaking and thinking clearly in financial terms and concepts. Without these skills it will be difficult for them to convey their thoughts and to understand what other managers are trying to communicate. When the failure to communicate occurs, a greater potential exists for something to go wrong. More likely than not, this failure will eventually affect the day-to-day operations of the nursing unit. Whether in a hospital, nursing home, or medical clinic, the nurse is the basic contact between patient and provider. Hence, the impact of financial matters on nursing services can ultimately affect the delivery of primary services.

Many nurse administrators are reluctant to upgrade their financial management skills. This can create a significant problem for them managerially. Financial management presents an entirely new set of terminology and concepts that nurse administrators are not exposed to in their clinical training. To many nurse administrators the terminology is unique and confusing, but actually the concepts themselves are based on logical models. A basic accounting framework is the foundation supporting many financial issues. It establishes an understandable methodology for thinking. This logic is easily comprehended once the rudimentary vocabulary and concepts are learned and the models that integrate the concepts are analyzed. Although not all nurse administrators want to become highly proficient in financial management skills, even a fundamental knowledge will help them better communicate to other managers and improve the management of the programs for which they are responsible.

A strong grounding in the terminology of financial management is a prerequisite to progressing to more advanced concepts and their application. Yet many people do not take the time required to reach a satisfactory understanding of basic terminology and concepts. To avoid this dilemma, Chapter 2 is devoted solely to defining and explaining financial concepts, statements, and reports. The very essence of this chapter is the vocabulary itself. By understanding and building on this terminology, the nurse administrator should become more proficient in thinking in financial terms and in communicating to other managers through a common language. Perhaps more than any other aspect of their ability to use financial management concepts, nurse administrators will be judged by their ability to speak and think in financial terms. Therefore it is critical to attain a solid grounding in this terminology to ensure that they are evaluated for their management capability rather than failure to communicate.

Considering the extensive effort that nurses allocate to learning nursing and medical terminology, it is clear that most have the capability to absorb financial management concepts and terminology. This may be the biggest hurdle in achieving skill in financial management—developing a receptive and positive mind-set for understanding and using the ideas. However, like any learning experiences, familiarization with financial terminology requires hard work as well as repeated application.

The biggest obstacle to this transfer is attaining competence in the basic vocabulary. Admittedly this is not always easy because there is nothing particularly glamorous about a balance sheet, income statement, or statement of changes in financial position. For nurse administrators, their personal challenge is to achieve a mind-set from which they can master financial terminology. Once this mind-set is attained, familiarization with financial concepts will be easier.

BASIC FINANCIAL TERMINOLOGY

Many of the financial statements and reports that nurse administrators have encountered are laden with terms that require definition. Additionally, certain standard statements and reports provide the foundation for financial management. This terminology and the statements are designed to convey an overall impression of the health care program or organization. The reports essentially present a profile of the financial health of the organization at one point in time, or over several periods of performance (e.g., fiscal years). This financial condition serves as a basis for decision making on the part of managers.

The Balance Sheet

The balance sheet is one of the three most important financial documents. The income statement and the statement of changes in financial position are usually acknowledged as the other critical financial reports. There may be other equally valuable documents, but this depends on the requirements of every health care organization. The balance sheet, income statement, and statement of changes in financial position are acknowledged in the business world as the primary reports necessary to assess the financial health of an organization. It must be remembered that health care organizations differ substantially from other business enterprises; consequently the content of these reports will also vary. However, the importance of the reports generally does not vary.

The peculiarities of the health field—notably third party reimbursement and an emphasis on patient utilization of services—may alter the relevance of documents, reports, or statements that support the three fundamental financial documents. Therefore, to fully understand the financial position of a health care organization it is usually necessary to assess utilization statistics in addition to the more traditional financial reports. These supplemental reports will be discussed after first reviewing the three basic reports. Remember that there is no ultimate or ideal set of financial statements. They all provide information for assessment of performance. It is up to the nurse administrator to become adept at reviewing *all* of the information and integrating it into an understandable whole that facilitates improved decision making.

In terms of the balance sheet, there are three fundamental forms of information conveyed—assets, liabilities, and fund balances. These three concepts are essential to understanding the *economic conditions* of the health care organization. The specific arrangement of assets, liabilities, and fund balances on a balance sheet is shown in Table 2–1. Notice that several concepts differentiate this balance sheet from that normally found for other corporations. This difference involves the historical characteristics of the health services field, notably the prevalence of nonprofit organizations and charitable contributions. These differences have been rapidly eroded and may ultimately have little impact on operations in the future.

Fund Accounting

In Table 2–1 a distinction is made between general funds (or nonrestricted funds) and restricted funds (or donor-restricted and endowment funds). This distinction captures a primary difference between health care organizations and business corporations. Nonprofit organizations like health care facilities are often recipients of funds from external sources that are used for special purposes. The donor may restrict the philanthropic gift (e.g., to restrict the investment to a building for a cancer center) and its use. In this case the assets are accounted for as donor-restricted funds. Alternatively the donor may provide funds to a general endowment allocated for unspecified purposes (although there are situations in which the endowment is restricted in its use). For example, half of the interest from the endowment fund might be targeted for research projects in the cancer center, while the remaining profit may be reinvested to keep the fund growing.

This differentiation in funds—general, donor-restricted, and endowment funds—results from the nonprofit nature of many health care organizations.

Table 2–1 Illustrated Balance Sheet

General Funds

Assets		
Cash		$ 4,000
Accounts Receivable[1]	50,000	
Less: Allowance for Uncollectibles	5,800	44,200
Inventory		7,500
Land, Buildings, and Equipment[2]	2,125,000	
Less: Accumulated Depreciation[3]	100,000	2,025,000
Board-designated Funds		50,000
TOTAL ASSETS		$2,130,700

Liabilities and Fund Balance		
Liabilities		
Accounts Payable		$ 48,000
Long-term Debt (Mortgage)		1,790,700
Precollected Revenue		78,000
Expenses Payable (Bank Loan)		14,000
Total Liabilities		1,930,700
Fund Liabilities and Fund Balance		200,000
TOTAL LIABILITIES AND FUND BALANCE		$2,130,700

Donor-Restricted Funds (Cancer Center)

Cash	$ 1,000	Accounts Payable	$ 2,000
Investments	35,000	Plant Fund Balance	204,000
Building and Equipment	170,000		
TOTAL ASSETS	$206,000	TOTAL LIABILITIES AND FUND BALANCE	$206,000

Endowment Fund

Cash	$ 2,000	Endowment	$225,000
Bonds	145,000		
Stock	78,000		
TOTAL ASSETS	$225,000	ENDOWMENT FUND BALANCE	$225,000

Note: For footnotes see section "Footnotes To Financial Statements" later in this chapter.

Whether for philanthropic or tax reasons, individuals have donated various assets to the organization. These funds must remain separated from normal (or general) operating assets. This accounting distinction is decidedly unique from the normal treatment of the balance sheet by business corporations. A corporation does not enjoy the tax advantages of the nonprofit organization and as a result is not required to distinguish among its sources of funds in this manner. However, the obvious trend in the health care field is increasingly toward the corporate model. There is substantial opportunity for this trend to continue since over 70 percent of all health care organizations are essentially nonprofit in orientation. The point is that fund accounting will remain a salient feature of financial balance sheets in the health field. But presently there are forces that increasingly make a health care organization's balance sheet comparable with corporate balance sheets.

The fundamental issue in fund accounting is to keep assets separated. An account or fund is primarily a convention for segregating assets and conveying that information to internal and external parties. The general fund is the only account for which net income is possible, because by definition income can be derived only from operations. This does not preclude earning (or losing) economic value on other assets such as those in the restricted funds. Depending on the extent to which the restricted funds are wisely invested there may be economic returns in the form of interest, dividends, stock gains (e.g., stock split), rent, or return on the sale of assets. There are also potential losses in the form of fees, bankrupt investments, and devaluation of investments. These losses must be accounted for (like the gains) in the adjustment of the restricted fund accounts. Normally this information is contained in the statement of changes in financial position, which must ultimately be reconciled with the balance sheet.

It should be noted that the restrictions accompanying an endowment, or specific purpose fund, are normally not provided as information on the balance sheet. This ancillary information may be useful in assessing the flexibility of a health care organization to meet financial crises, but such information only complicates assessing the overall financial profile of the organization. Normally the information on endowment restrictions is listed in notes that accompany the financial statement.

Unless the gift or endowment has been specified as restricted for a certain use, the board of trustees of an organization may invoke its privilege of using the gift or its interest (or other economic return) for the well-being of the organization. The actual endowment, or principal, is seldom used for operating purposes—this action would neglect the fiduciary responsibilities of the board. Only in emergencies is the endowment drawn down (i.e., expended), and only if the funds are unrestricted. A more prevalent option is to employ the earnings on the principal to fund current operations.

Balance Sheet Terminology

The terminology in Table 2–2 is often found on balance sheets and associated financial statements. It is essential that nurse administrators develop a working familiarity with this terminology in order to converse with other health care managers. Again, effectiveness in financial management begins with a firm understanding of the key terms and concepts.

Although the illustrated balance sheet in Table 2–1 does indicate separate categories for general funds, donor-restricted funds, and the endowment fund, it should be recognized that the nature of accounting for health care organizations is gradually changing. Certainly increasing corporate involvement in the health field is partly responsible for these changes. The practical translation of corporate involvement in the health field is a change in financial reports toward formats more often used in other businesses.

Despite the fact that nonprofit health care organizations (and others) will continue to have balance sheets that identify separate funds, the extent of fund accounting may soon diminish as philanthropy changes and donors are encouraged not to over restrict contributions. However, in an environment that is resource-constrained, it is probable that health care organizations will continue to seek contributions. Thus, fund accounting may continue to provide the necessary legal and management control guidelines relevant to a pluralistic funding environment (e.g., philanthropy, private pay, third party reimbursement, corporate invest-ment, and so forth).

The Statement of Revenues and Expenses

Corporations report their diverse sources of income on an income statement; the equivalent income statement used in the health care field is called the statement of revenues and expenses. The difference between these two is the need to retain a nonprofit orientation. Income implies profit. Traditionally the health care field has not supported profit making as an ethically legitimate goal. This bias may result from the dominant ethics of the medical profession, which views quality of care as the preeminent goal of health care providers. Consideration was seldom given to economic surplus because attention was directed toward delivering the highest quality of care attainable. Profit under this ethic was superfluous and misdirected.

Today health care organizations are vitally aware of the need to balance quality and costs. Resources are constrained and it is less feasible to sacrifice financial solvency for quality of care. Nonprofit organizations themselves must think of an acceptable accounting rate of return that permits enough surplus from operations to maintain the equity position of the health care organization. For all of these reasons, nurse administrators will increasingly discover income statements, as

Table 2–2 Financial Statement Terminology

Term	Definition	Illustrations
Asset	A resource having exchange or economic value	Surgery skills of a physician; nursing home beds; nursing supplies
Fixed Asset	An asset that is assessed a long economic life (i.e., will retain usefulness for more than one year)	Hospital buildings; a lithotripter; a parking structure; land
Liquid Asset or Current Asset	An asset that is in negotiable form or could easily be converted into negotiable form within one year	Cash; patient accounts receivable; marketable securities (e.g., stock in a corporation)
Cash	Money	A demand deposit of $1,000; petty cash of $43.71
Accounts Receivable	A current asset that consists of amounts or payments due the organization as a result of services or products provided	Patient charges for bypass surgery that have not been paid; usually this represents the delay necessary to process and file claims for payment from third parties
Allowance for Uncollectibles	An adjustment to accounts receivable that reflects the amount of free (or charitable) care provided by the organization or the extent of bad debts (Many third party payers will pay only a portion of bad debts and charitable care.)	Unpaid accounts for 53 patients who have signed a preadmission agreement to cover their expenses personally due to the lack of insurance coverage (After treatment, the patients refused to pay.)
Inventory	A current asset consisting of supplies necessary to support the provision of services or products	Nursing supplies; pharmaceuticals; food products; maintenance supplies
Accumulated Depreciation	A normal expense of doing business that reflects the deterioration of plant and equipment (Fixed assets often wear out from use; thus their value decreases—this is an anticipated aspect of using assets.)	Aging of a hospital wing (i.e., 20 years of use); 40,000 scans completed on a CAT scanner

Board-Designated Funds	Funds donated to a health care organization for use at the discretion of the board (These funds have no other restrictions, otherwise they would be classified as donor-restricted funds or as endowments.)	A $10,000 donation to the board to use as it deems appropriate in covering the expenses of a hospital
Liabilities	A category of financial responsibilities and debts that have resulted from current operations and from investment in fixed assets necessary to perform services or produce products	$5,376 owed to a linen supply company for new linen; $2 million loan from the bank to build a new wing on a nursing home
Accounts Payable	Short-term debts incurred in the provision of services or products	Bills for utilities; bills for new food supplies or pharmaceuticals
Long-Term Debt	Debt that is typically paid over a period greater than one year (This debt is usually incurred in order to fund assets with a long fixed life as opposed to funding short-term operations.)	$1.5 million dollar mortgage to construct a new clinic
Precollected Revenue	Revenue that is collected before products or services are delivered	$250,000 in prepaid premiums for a health maintenance organization; $100,000 in prospective payments from a third party (which may later be retrospectively adjusted)
Expenses Payable	Special expenses that may not fit in the short-term or long-term debt categories, for example, a two-year loan to buffer the cash needs of a facility	Bank loan of $50,000 payable over 24 months at an interest rate of 13.325%

opposed to statements of revenues and expenses, being used in their organizations. The fact that terminology and accepted practice have changed the income statement is not an academic point. It reflects the ongoing changes taking place in financial management practices of health care organizations. It therefore alerts nurse administrators about the need to concentrate on economic efficiency and profitability. More health care organizations are being managed with the bottom line—income—clearly in mind.

One of the primary purposes underlying the statement of revenues and expenses is to provide a measure of how well an organization is doing in accomplishing its goals. The nonprofit organization has normally been concerned with providing services without concern for an economic surplus. Nonetheless, nonprofit organizations use the statement of revenues and expenses to take the pulse of their performance. Among other questions, they may seek to answer many of the following issues by examining their statements of revenues and expenses:

- Which third parties are predominantly funding operations?
- To what extent are private pay patients subsidizing other patients?
- Is there a dangerous imbalance in the sources of revenue (i.e., overreliance on one main source)?
- What is the financial performance of specific programs—are more expenses being incurred than revenues obtained?
- What trends exist in the balance of revenues and expenses (i.e., are expenses consistently higher than revenues, which may therefore affect long-run survivability)?
- Has too much surplus been earned, which suggests either expanding service benefits or reducing prices?
- What are the major expense categories and what policies and practices are being implemented to control expenses?
- Are any expense areas rising more rapidly than others and therefore need priority attention?
- What are the implications of surplus or negative earning for the long-run financial solvency of the organization?

Clearly these questions require significant analysis of the statement of revenues and expenses not only in one year but over several years as well. It is this sort of analysis that helps managers understand where their organizations have been and where they are going. A wealth of information is contained in the statement of revenues and expenses; it is merely a matter of taking enough time to analyze the information and trends.

As far as for-profit health care corporations are concerned, the preceding questions are also highly relevant to their examination of performance. For-profit corporations should not be any more obsessed with performance than nonprofit organizations. Both should be vitally interested in how they are performing, not only in analyzing sources of revenue but also in critically reviewing categories of expenditures. The point is that managers, such as nurse administrators, must use statements of revenues and expenses (or income statements) for monitoring performance.

Once they analyze the financial data, they are in a position to alter the structure and process of operations accordingly. This applies especially to the for-profit organization that may interpret high levels of profit or income as indicating exemplary performance. True, high net income does suggest excellent performance. However, it is critical that all health care managers remember that performance can always be improved. Thus it is necessary to go beyond the bottom line in analyzing the specific components of performance. This analysis should be guided by the questions noted above.

The statement of revenues and expenses is a very valuable management tool if nursing administrators and other managers want it to be important. Not only can it act as a barometer on performance, it can also be used to detect situations that require more management attention. From the nurse administrator's perspective, this concept is vitally important. It allows the organization to focus accurately on the real causes of financial problems rather than just infer suspicions.

For example, a nurse administrator may be under pressure from a hospital administrator because department salary expenses are so high relative to other departments. An appraisal of the last three statements of revenues and expenses may suggest an entirely different perspective. Assume the data shown in Table 2–3. Although nursing expenses are far higher in total magnitude than any of the other expense categories, the nursing department may not deserve the hospital administrator's specially focused concern. The analysis of expense trends indicates that the percentage increases (rounded) are much lower for nursing than for either dietary or administration. At issue is the proportionate increase in expenses. Dietary and administration have increased at a much higher rate than nursing. Therefore it is essential that management direct its attention to cost control in these two areas.

Similarly, it should be noted that housekeeping has maintained the lowest rate of percentage increase. The question is why? If there is an answer to this question

Table 2–3 A Yearly Analysis of Departmental Performance Trends

		Performance Trends			
	1986	% Change 1985–1986	1985	% Change 1984–1985	1984
Nursing	$676,714	+13	$600,008	+16	$518,764
Dietary	76,060	+24	61,339	+22	50,235
Housekeeping	85,313	+ 9	78,287	+ 8	72,166
Administration	74,333	+16	64,255	+28	50,100

that can be transferred to the other departments, then the organization as a whole can benefit. When other departments such as nursing use housekeeping as a comparative base, nursing appears to have excessive increases in expenses. However, the housekeeping department may be able to keep expenses low because there is an oversupply of unskilled employees willing to take jobs in housekeeping. Nursing may be searching for applicants to fill vacant positions. The shortage of applicants means few filled positions, higher overall staffing costs, and higher overtime expenses. It is the visual display of the figures themselves that allows further analysis.

An example of a statement of revenues and expenses is shown in Table 2–4. Remember that it differs from the income statement mainly in the fact that there is no net income to report. There may be a net increase in the fund balance if revenues actually do exceed expenses. However, it is the treatment of the surplus that gives significance to the for-profit ownership status of the health care organization. Net income is available for distribution to shareholders in the for-profit corporation, whereas a net increase in fund balances results where revenues exceed expenses in a nonprofit organization.

Table 2–4 Illustrated Statement of Revenues and Expenses

Patient Care Revenues	$175,434
Adjustment for Allowances and Uncollected Accounts	(42,111)
Net Patient Care Revenue	$133,323
Other Operating Revenue	18,787
Total Operating Revenue	$152,110
Operating Expenses	
Nursing	$ 54,313
Dietary	20,111
Housekeeping	14,784
Administration and General	19,008
Depreciation	15,470
Total Operating Expenses	$123,686
Net Operating Revenue	28,424
Nonoperating Revenue	1,576
Excess of Revenues Over Expenses (Loss) or Net Increase in Fund Balance	$ 30,000

As the title implies, there are two major categories of information shown in Table 2–4—sources of revenue and sources of expenses. There are variations in how much detail each of the revenue and expense categories will actually display. For example, the patient service revenue category may include specification of the relative contribution by key third party payers (e.g., Medicare, Medicaid, self-pay, commercial carrier, and others); and delineation of funds received from local, state, or federal grants and contracts (*for patient care*), donations for patient care, or other sources. Alternatively, the convention of lumping all payers together may be used especially where one dominant third party payer is involved in funding the majority of operations. Greater detail can be given in notes and/or additional appended statements when clarification is needed.

It may also be appropriate to identify the sources of other operating revenues if those sources are numerous (e.g., vending machines, unrestricted investments, gift shops, parking, unrestricted gifts, unrestricted endowments, or other income from programs that support patient care but may also derive income by selling services/products—a prevalent example might be a shared laundry service). In these cases a separate category should be established.

It is essential to recognize that the excess of revenue over expenses could just as well be a loss, depending on how well the organization is managed. In these cases the loss is reported in parentheses to indicate the loss. Note that adjustments are also indicated in parentheses. This signifies a deduction or subtraction. Finally, it should also be pointed out that in the case of a for-profit corporation the entry for the excess of revenue over expenses will simply be replaced by the term "net income (loss)."

Revenue and Expenses Terminology

The terminology in Table 2–5 is often found on income statements, statements of revenues and expenses, and related financial statements. As with the balance sheet terminology it is essential that nurse administrators develop a working capability with this terminology. These terms are the basis for communicating with other financially oriented managers and the building blocks upon which financial management is founded. By developing this familiarity it will be possible to both think and speak along the same lines as other health care managers.

Although knowledge of these terms and concepts is a helpful step in understanding the operations of a health care facility, it is the *use* of the income statement (or statement of revenues and expenses) that has the most meaning. There is no substitute for analysis that compares one expense (revenue) category with another over a period of time. However, the timing of a given expense or revenue may confound such comparisons. This mixing of revenues and expenses from one time period to another is inevitable and should not present an obstacle to understanding

Table 2–5 Revenue and Expenses Terminology

Term	Definition	Illustrations
Patient Care Revenues	Revenues received for delivery of services and products (or packages of care) to patients (These revenues are reported at a gross level, i.e., all services at their respective charges for those services.)	$1,239 received from Blue Cross for two days hospital care, $124 for an intravenous pyelogram
Adjustments	Adjustments to gross revenues to reflect deductions (The prevalent deductions include allowances for charity, bad debts [uncollected accounts], and contractual allowances, i.e., an agreement with a third party to provide a special discount.)	$5,432 loss from a patient who died with no relatives; an agreement to provide a 3% discount to all patients of Ingenious Insurance Company; $125,000 in free care given to medically indigent patients
Other Operating Revenue	Revenues derived from daily operations of the health care organization that are not related to direct patient care (These revenues may result from indirect patient care or from supporting programs that derive a portion of their income from external sales of products and services, but for which they are mainly supporting of the main organization.) May also include revenues from education and research programs	Cafeteria sales to staff and the public; revenues from patient amenities (e.g., television and telephone); gift shop and newsstand sales; fees from registrants in a parent education program
Total Operating Revenue	All patient care and other operating revenues less any deductions for discounts or allowances	The sum total of revenues against which all expenses must be balanced
Operating Expenses	Expenses incurred when conducting business, i.e., providing services (These expenses may be broken down to include some or all of the following functional areas: nursing, laboratory, x-ray, dietary, administrative and general housekeeping maintenance, property, and patient care. They are often categorized to include	Depreciation on a nursing home; expenses associated with the nursing and laboratory departments

	the following: interest, depreciation, payroll [i.e., salaries and wages], supplies, and insurance. Unlike other business organizations, interest is seen as an operating expense.)	
Net Operating Revenue	A financial outcome from the process of delivering services that signifies the profitability of operations	The balance of total operating revenues after deducting total operating expenses
Nonoperating Revenue	Revenue derived from sources other than current operations (These revenues normally include nonrestricted donations, net sales of equipment and fixed assets, or donated assets.)	A grant of $10,000 from a donor to be applied to general operations; donation of 12 wheelchairs by the women's auxiliary of a hospital
Net Income (Excess of Revenues over Expenses)	The surplus (or loss) that results from current operations and donations	The bottom-line figure on the income statement

how an organization performs. The basic problem in health care organizations is that revenues will usually be received well after services have been delivered. Thus expenses incurred in delivering services will not match with revenues. There is no single conclusion possible about the precise lag in receipt of revenues—each organization's receipts will vary according to its patient/payer mix.

A number of accounting and mathematical conventions have been created to resolve this problem in unmatched revenues and expenses. In the case of forecasting either revenues or expenses, the assumptions underlying the mathematical models can easily be incorporated into the model of an organization. The same is true for models that associate the revenues and expenses. From a decision-making perspective, it is important to remember that there is a lag between when expenses are incurred and when revenues are received. Ultimately the lag can lead to a misinterpretation of cause and effect unless it is accounted for in the decision-making analysis.

For example, an advertising expenditure (an administrative and general expense) may not produce tangible increases in revenue for several months. First, the patients must respond to the promotion. It is clear that patients will generally wait until they have a symptom that can be resolved through the advertised service. Such a condition may take months or years to develop. Second, the care must be billed to the third party (assuming that patients are covered by insurance), and then the third party must process payment. It should be apparent that revenues and expenses seldom match. Therefore, avoid such assumptions when interpreting data and instead seek to ascertain precisely the length of lag between when services are delivered—expenses incurred—and when revenues are received.

Statement of Changes in Fund Balances

The third essential financial statement is concerned with how fund balances have changed over a fiscal year or period due to current operations, philanthropy, fund-raising, and other external events that ultimately influence fund balances. The for-profit equivalent of the statement of changes in fund balances is known as the statement of changes in financial position. The difference between the two is essentially due to fund accounting.

The purpose of the statement of changes in fund balances is to reconcile the balance sheet with the statement of revenues and expenses. The actual effect of the statement of revenues and expenses is to add or delete funds from a given balance sheet. The statement of changes in fund balance helps clarify key transactions that lead to variations between balance sheets. It summarizes the major changes in financial position of the organization between periods. The statement of changes in financial position is therefore invaluable in helping managers and analysts determine whether the financial strength (or weakness) of an organization is a result of current operations or manipulations of fixed assets.

The statement of changes in fund balances is an important tool for determining how well assets and operations are managed. If cost control and judicious cash flow management are implemented without significant changes in revenue flows, an organization may be able to fund long-term debt internally and prepare for acquisition of new capital assets. This ability to service debt (i.e., pay monthly principal and interest) from current operations has long been a problem in the capital structure of organizations. Many health care organizations have a history of spending more than they should. This has tremendous implications for management of fixed assets. Normally, philanthropy or government grants were used to balance the need between operations and capital assets. Current funds went to current operations and services with little set aside for servicing debt. These policies have been changed due to diminishing governmental funds and declining philanthropy.

Tax-free revenue bonds replaced philanthropy and government funds in providing capital to health care organizations. When this occurred, the ability to pay for the interest and principal associated with borrowed capital became important. The end result is that current operations must be increasingly managed to resolve a health care organization's capital needs. The statement of changes in fund balances provides direct evidence on management effectiveness in this regard. When management relies on debt to fund either current operations or fixed assets there will be significant ramifications for control. Either costs are controlled or revenues are raised in order to pay for this debt. The addition of debt does not occur in a vacuum—most facilities already have an existing debt structure. Thus, management must plan to break the descending spiral of operating beyond available means. Once such a spiral begins, it is very difficult to exit. The statement of changes in fund balances will show this within a limited number of reporting periods.

Changes in Fund Balances Terminology

The terminology associated with the statement of changes in fund balances has already been explained in depth for the balance sheet and the statement of revenues over expenses. However, it is useful to go through a statement in order to interpret the changes in fund balances. In this manner it will be possible to determine how management acquired funds and used them during the year. In order to create a statement of changes in fund balances it is necessary to have two fiscal reports for balance sheets and income statements. A two-year profile is presented in Table 2–6, which provides an additional year's data to that already displayed in Tables 2–1 and 2–4.

To facilitate understanding the changes in performance, Table 2–6 assumes that neither the donor-restricted fund nor the endowment fund in Table 2–1 changed in this time period. This assumption permits an undistracted focus on the general operations (i.e., general funds) of the organization. Furthermore, Table 2–6 has condensed the reporting of balance sheet and income statement items in order to direct attention to the significant alterations in the acquisition and disposal of funds.

Table 2–7 illustrates the calculation of changes in balance sheet accounts. This is the beginning from which the statement of changes in fund balances is initiated. Each change in the balance sheet accounts is classified as a source or a use. In some instances there are no changes in the accounts; hence, they are not shown in Table 2–7. Additionally, the summary accounts (e.g., total assets) are not shown because if they were incorporated in the calculations, they would have been entered twice, resulting in double accounting for some items.

The changes in the balance sheet accounts can be used to formulate the statement of changes in fund balances shown in Table 2–8. The approach shown in Table 2–8 is to interpret the use of funds as alterations in working capital that must be combined with changes in nonworking capital. During the latest fiscal year the organization had two nonworking capital sources of funds that totaled $40,000. Net income was derived at a level of $30,000 and depreciation totaled $10,000. These funds were offset by a decrease in net working capital as shown in Table 2–8.

Table 2-6 Two-Year Profile of Financial Performance

Assets	Year 1995	Year 1994
Cash	$ 4,000	$ 3,500
Accounts Receivable	50,000	52,000
Less: Allowances	5,800	5,800
Net Accounts Receivable	48,200	49,700
Inventory	7,500	7,000
Total Current Assets	55,700	56,700
Land, Buildings, and Equipment	2,125,000	2,100,000
Less: Accumulated Depreciation	100,000	90,000
Total Fixed Assets	2,025,000	2,010,000
Board-Designated Funds	50,000	50,000
TOTAL ASSETS	$2,130,700	$2,116,700
Liabilities and Fund Balance		
Accounts Payable	$ 48,000	$ 38,000
Long-Term Debt	1,790,700	1,790,700
Precollected Revenue	78,000	78,000
Expenses Payable	14,000	10,000
Total Liabilities	1,930,700	1,916,700
Fund Balance	200,000	200,000
TOTAL LIABILITIES AND FUND BALANCE	$2,130,700	2,116,700

	Year 1995	Year 1994
Revenues		
Patient Care	$175,434	$164,211
Less: Adjustments	42,111	37,674
Net Patient Care	133,323	126,537
Other Operating Revenue	18,787	16,139
Total Operating Revenue	152,110	142,676
Expenses		
Nursing	$ 54,313	$ 49,617
Dietary	20,111	19,878
Housekeeping	14,784	15,675
Administration and General	19,008	25,499
Depreciation	15,470	15,000
Total Operating Expenses	123,686	125,669
Net Operating Revenue	28,424	17,007
Nonoperating Revenue	1,576	1,234
NET INCOME	$ 30,000	$ 18,241

Table 2–7 Changes in Balance Sheet Accounts

	Year 1995	Year 1994	Change Source	Use
Cash	$ 4,000	$ 3,500		$ 500
Accounts Receivable	50,000	52,000	$ 2,000	
Inventory	7,500	7,000		500
Land, Buildings, and Equipment	2,125,000	2,100,000		25,000
Accumulated Depreciation	100,000	90,000	10,000	
Accounts Payable	48,000	38,000	10,000	
Expenses Payable	14,000	10,000	4,000	
			$26,000	$26,000

Table 2–8 Statement of Changes in Fund Balances

Sources of Funds
Net Income (1995)	$30,000
Depreciation	10,000
Total Nonworking Capital Sources	40,000
Decrease in Net Working Capital	(15,000)
TOTAL SOURCES	$25,000

Uses of Funds
Increase in Fixed Assets (Land, Buildings, and Equipment)	$25,000
TOTAL USES	$25,000

Analysis of Changes in Working Capital
Increase (Decrease) in Current Assets
Cash	$ 500
Accounts Receivable	(2,000)
Inventory	500
Net Decrease in Current Assets	($1,000)

Increase (Decrease) in Current Liabilities
Accounts Payable	$10,000
Expenses Payable	4,000
Net Increases in Current Liabilities	$14,000
Decrease in Net Working Capital	$15,000

The analysis of changes in working capital indicates that there was a net decrease in current assets of $1,000. Although actual cash and the value of the inventory each increased $500, accounts receivable declined $2,000. Added to this decrease in current assets is a net increase in current liabilities. Accounts payable rose by $10,000 and expenses payable increased $4,000. Together, the net decrease in current assets ($1,000) plus the net increase in current liabilities ($14,000) results in a total decrease in working capital of $15,000. Added to the nonworking capital sources of funds, the decrease in working capital lowers available funds to $25,000 (i.e., $40,000 − $15,000). The funds were used to increase fixed assets by $25,000.

Table 2–8 provides a convenient summary of the source and use of funds. This statement of changes in fund balances suggests that the nonworking capital sources helped to fund the acquisition of a fixed asset valued at $25,000. The sources were also allocated to cover current liabilities, notably a rise in accounts payable and expenses payable (i.e., a loan). The data suggest that the fixed asset was partially funded through internal operations, but a supplement of $4,000 was also needed in the form of a short-term loan.

As this examination of the statement of changes in fund balance suggests, only an initial map is presented to provide direction through analyses of financial performance. It serves as a useful method for ascertaining the overall efficiency of capital use. It can also determine the effectiveness of management decisions such as financial commitments in the acquisition of assets. But this is only a beginning. Further exploration depends on asking the right questions, guided by the entries to the statement of changes in fund balances.

FOOTNOTES TO FINANCIAL STATEMENTS

Many financial statements are accompanied by footnotes that further explain entries on the statements. The purpose is usually to provide clarification or additional detail that would otherwise confuse the overall summary presented by the financial statement. For example, there are three footnotes in Table 2–1. The following explanations may represent the information conveyed in these footnotes:

Note 1: Third Party Receivables
Reimbursement of costs related to patient care administered under the Medicaid and Medicare programs is subject to examination by reimbursement agencies who have analyzed and made final settlement on cost reports through the prior fiscal period. Currently, the organization is due $23,764 from these third parties.

Note 2: Equipment
Purchased equipment is recorded at acquisition cost and contributed equipment is recorded at fair value at the date of contribution.

Note 3: Depreciation
Plant and equipment are depreciated using the straight-line method over the estimated useful lives of the assets. The original costs, accumulated depreciation, and net book value of the various classes of plant and equipment follow:

	Original Cost or Value	Accumulated Depreciation	Net Book Value
Buildings	2,000,000	75,000	1,925,000
Equipment	100,000	25,000	75,000
	2,100,000	100,000	2,000,000

As these notes suggest, more information is provided with which to make a fair and accurate assessment of the financial status of the organization.

SUPPORTING CONCEPTS

The balance sheet, income statement, and statement of changes in financial position are the fundamental reports upon which financial management practices are based. However, these reports are only a prelude to the diversity of concepts and reporting conventions used by managers to understand and control operations. From the perspective of nurse administrators, this foundation is critical to their ability to work with other health care managers. It is also essential that they progress beyond these basics toward more advanced concepts. A key ingredient in facilitating this growth is a working knowledge of supporting financial management concepts. These ideas and techniques are prerequisites for translating business-oriented financial reports to the health care context. Several ideas are important in this regard.

Contractual Allowances

Allowances to gross patient revenues have to be made when patients are unable or unwilling to pay their bills. Third party payers are not simply going to assume responsibility for the cost of these items. Health care organizations have to reach an agreement with third parties on what allowances will be covered by contracts. These allowances will be combined with various adjustments or discounts that the hospital agrees to. For example, a health maintenance organization may decide to establish a discount for a certain employer group. This allowance must be adjusted during the final tally of patient revenues. It may also be an allowance that should be incorporated into the calculation of charges for other third party payers.

The rationale for contractual allowances is easy to understand. Services that are rendered must be paid by someone at some point. Hospitals naturally prefer to have all of their costs covered. Third party payers prefer to cover only those costs that represent the delivery of services to their enrollees. The cost shifting that occurs when rates do not match costs is a prevalent strategy among hospitals to recover expenditures. The self-paying patient often experiences the brunt of this cost shifting. The third party payer is in a better position to negotiate a discount or contractual allowance to avoid assuming a greater responsibility for added costs.

Alternatively, services that are provided at a discounted rate may also represent a contractual allowance of distinct importance. These services are often discounted in order to market care to a specific population group. Allowances are usually contractually determined in advance. They must ultimately be accounted for on the books of the health care organization. These costs are susceptible to being shifted to other payers; naturally third party payers monitor such attempts very closely. As a result, health care organizations are forced to absorb the cost, raise productivity to cover the cost, or transfer the cost to willing third parties (e.g., self-paying patients or fractionated commercial insurers who may have little bargaining power).

Depreciation

One of the most misunderstood financial concepts is the depreciation of land, plant, and equipment. The reason for this misunderstanding probably stems from the fact that *depreciation is an allowable expense* or deduction for income tax purposes. However, it is not a cash expense; that is, the health care facility does not pay direct out-of-pocket cash resources to cover the expense. This is where the confusion enters because health care managers may have difficulty conceiving of expenses that do not involve a monetary transaction. How can an expense be an expense if the health care organization does not pay directly for goods, services, or capital assets?

The answer is found in the long-run nature of the investments. Plant and major equipment are financed over long periods of time because they are durable assets that last for years. However, each year takes a toll on plant and equipment—physical items eventually wear out or become too dated to perform effectively. This process of decreasing value over time is known as depreciation. An accounting convention is used to adjust the books of a corporation for this deterioration. The depreciation is spread over as many years as the plant or equipment is normally perceived to be a productive asset. Land generally does not depreciate in value, although there are cases where this is possible given urban decay or other community and geographical changes that alter the value of land. Land is more likely to be depleted (i.e., in terms of natural resources).

Authorities often do not agree on how to calculate depreciation. For some assets depreciation occurs most extensively in the initial years. A lithotripter to treat kidney stones is just such an asset. Given the rapid change in technology, a lithotripter may have a feasible economic life of four years, even though it could be used over a ten-year period. Its technological obsolescence is reached before its physical obsolescence. On the other hand, a hospital building deteriorates at a relatively constant rate. Thus, its depreciation should be treated as a constant amount with the level in one year the same as the next. This idea of variability in depreciation is easy to comprehend and calculate. There are several prevalent techniques for calculating depreciation.

The point of contention that surrounds depreciation involves the payment of taxes. If an accelerated method of computing depreciation is used, then the expenses of depreciation will be higher in the initial years of an asset. Consequently, less tax is paid in those early years. This has the net effect of delaying payment of taxes. Lower tax payments mean that current funds can be invested to obtain a higher return or at least higher earnings in the short run. The only consideration that invalidates this conclusion is the tax rate. If taxes are expected to rise in the future this strategy is questionable; if the tax rate is expected to decrease in the future the strategy becomes increasingly viable.

The tax advantages can be easily understood by analyzing the methods of computing depreciation. The straight-line method of calculating depreciation relaxes the assumptions about the variability of depreciation over the life of an asset. It is assumed that the level of depreciation from one year to the next is equal. Therefore, the cost of the asset is divided by the number of years of its useful life after adjusting for any salvage value:

Straight-Line Depreciation

Value of Asset	= $100,000
Useful Life	= 7 years
Salvage Value at End of Life	= $13,000
Yearly Depreciation	$= \dfrac{\$100,000 - \$13,000}{7} = \$12,428.57$

At the end of 7 years, the amount of depreciation (7 × $12,428.57) will equal the value of the asset minus any salvage value. An expense of $12,428.57 is recorded each year under this methodology. Note that the total investment may have occurred in the first year—therefore there is no cash expense each year unless the terms of financing were arranged in that manner. In any case, by accounting for depreciation the financing issue is kept separate from the expense issue.

The sum-of-years-digits is another prevalent method for calculating depreciation. Compared with straight-line depreciation it is an accelerated method for calculating depreciation expenses. Each year's depreciation is calculated as a fraction of the number of years of remaining life, which are summed. Since the fraction becomes smaller with each passing year, it is apparent that the level of depreciation actually expended is much higher in the first few years. The tax advantages of this method can be very substantial because it accelerates the expenses that can be deducted in the initial years:

Sum-of-Years-Digits

Value of Asset   = $100,000
Useful Life   = 7 years
Salvage Value at End of Life = $13,000
Sum of Useful Years   = 7 + 6 + 5 + 4 + 3 + 2 + 1 = 28 years

Year		Amount of Depreciation
1	$(7 \div 28) \times (\$100,000 - \$13,000) =$	$21,750.00
2	$(6 \div 28) \times (\$100,000 - \$13,000) =$	18,270.00
3	$(5 \div 28) \times (\$100,000 - \$13,000) =$	15,660.00
4	$(4 \div 28) \times (\$100,000 - \$13,000) =$	12,180.00
5	$(3 \div 28) \times (\$100,000 - \$13,000) =$	9,570.00
6	$(2 \div 28) \times (\$100,000 - \$13,000) =$	6,090.00
7	$(1 \div 28) \times (\$100,000 - \$13,000) =$	3,480.00
	TOTAL =	$87,000.00

As the preceding figures indicate, there is much more depreciation accounted for in the first year ($21,750) than in the seventh year ($3,480). Compared with the straight-line method, there is an additional expense of $9,321.43 ($21,750 − $12,428.57 = $9,321.43) that can be taken in the first year to reduce taxes. The disadvantage comes at the end of the asset's life.

A third popular method of calculating depreciation is the double declining balance, another accelerated method. It is based on the half-life of the asset. The initial amount to be depreciated in the first year is divided by the number of years of life and then divided by two. All other years represent one-half of the total years of useful life. This method is based on historical cost, rather than cost less salvage value.

Double Declining Balance

Value of Asset = $100,000
Useful Life   = 7 years

Year	Depreciation Amount	Total Depreciation
1	28,571.43	28,571.43
2	20,408.16	48,979.59
3	14,577.26	63,556.85
4	10,412.33	73,969.18
5	7,437.35	81,406.56
6	5,312.41	86,718.97
7	3,794.58	90,513.55

As the total depreciation figures for the double declining balance suggest, a much higher rate of depreciation can be achieved than for either the straight-line or sum-of-years-digits in the first years.

The selection of an accounting method for depreciation formerly was a seriously contested issue, just as the ability to declare depreciation as an expense was a challenge for hospitals some years ago. These issues are fairly well resolved at this point in terms of costing-out depreciation as a legitimate expense. Depending on the third party, however, there may still be an issue about the use of accelerated depreciation and the basis for the depreciation (i.e., historical costs versus market or replacement costs). The best advice is to remain in close contact with third parties in negotiating these issues. Although nurse administrators may not be directly involved in such negotiations, their organization's accounting staff members may need guidance in terms of ascertaining a rationale for selecting a depreciation method or historical cost treatment.

Charity and Bad Debts

By law, the promotion of health is held to be a charitable purpose, a fact that deserves special consideration by the financial manager. The fact that health care organizations provide health care services, however, does not remove their inherent responsibilities for deriving net profits. In most hospitals, for example, there has traditionally been a greater problem with providing excessive charity care than with providing too little. This situation may be changing. A greater for-profit orientation by the health field is continually driving down the incentive to offer charitable care. This will certainly be one of the most relevant issues in the future of health care organizations. Who should receive free care and how much should be provided by any given health facility are salient questions that must be answered.

All hospitals hold a public trust even if they are chartered to operate for profit. Thus, they must ascertain their level of charitable care despite the fact that they may have made substantial profits. To some extent this attitude of tolerance for charitable care transfers over to the issue of bad debts. In the past, bad debts were more easily forgotten due to subsidizing by third party payers. These attitudes and practices reflect a bygone era that tolerated such inefficiencies in health care. A consistent and rigorous policy for managing bad debts and charitable care is now needed by every health care organization.

The nurse administrator's role in resolving problems of charitable care or bad debts may seem minor on the surface. After all, the nurse does not determine who or who will not be accorded free care. Nor does he/she assume the business risk when patients have been admitted. However, the nurse administrator needs guidance from the policy level. At some point, each organization must decide how much charitable care will be given. There is also an important realization that *each* employee has a responsibility to help the health care organization attain effective performance. In this regard nurse administrators may help provide input on determining the amount of free care to be delivered. For example, they can specify how resource-intensive are charitable care patients compared with paying patients. Such facts may be useful during formation of policies.

The Accrual Concept

Health care organizations face the dilemma of when to account for transactions on their books, just as any other business organization must decide when a transaction has occurred. With small corporations and health care facilities there is a tendency to account for transactions on the basis of exchanges in cash. This so-called cash accounting is a convenient mechanism for controlling the flow of cash. Many public and large private organizations have used such methods until relatively recently. For example, if a hospital borrows $2,500,000 to build a clinic it has incurred a liability of $2,500,000 and has increased its funds by $2,500,000. However, until those funds are invested in construction there is no actual change in the fund (or equity) balance.

To remedy this problem many health care organizations are now using the accrual concept. Accordingly, a transaction is reported on financial statements only if it affects equity (which in turn affects income). The most prevalent manner in which operations affect equity is through consumption of resources. Thus, the accrual concept measures the change in equity even though there may be no net effect on cash. This issue is relevant to nurse administrators in the sense that they must ascertain which accounting system (i.e., cash or accrual basis) is employed by their organization. There are distinct advantages to the accrual system, especially the accuracy in portraying changes in the asset base of the organization. The more complete profile of financial status provided by the accrual system suggests that it is a superior method of reporting operations.

The cash basis of accounting records revenues when they are received and expenses when they are paid. The cash basis recognizes only an exchange of cash. Under the accrual system, obligations are recorded when they are incurred rather than when a cash transaction occurs. If the cash basis is used for accounting, it is possible to distort the true status of an organization's financial position because debts and receivables will not be recorded. Consider the balance sheet for a nursing home under the cash basis:

Assets	
Cash	$1,100,000
TOTAL ASSETS	$1,100,000
Equity	
Fund Balance	$1,100,000
TOTAL EQUITY	$1,100,000

At the end of the fiscal period only the cash on hand has been recorded. It is balanced by equity. If the accrual method of accounting is used an entirely different profile emerges:

Assets	
Cash	$1,100,000
Accounts Receivable	2,400,000
Inventory	800,000
TOTAL ASSETS	$4,300,000
Equity	
Accounts Payable	$1,200,000
Note Payable	2,000,000
Fund Balance	1,100,000
TOTAL EQUITY	$4,300,000

Notice how much additional information is available with the accrual approach. It is apparent that a substantial level of patient care has been delivered for which payment has not been received (i.e., $2,400,000 of accounts receivable). Furthermore, the nursing home has accumulated $800,000 in inventory of dietary, housekeeping, nursing, and related supplies. At the same time, the assets are offset by accounts payable for expenses in delivering care that have not been paid. Similarly, it is apparent that the nursing home has a $2,000,000 note that must be paid. In sum, the accrual method of accounting provides the most detailed and accurate portrayal of an organization's financial status.

Uniform Reporting

Uniform reporting normally pertains to reporting financial and utilization data to various regulatory and reimbursement agencies. Usually there are regulations that require health care organizations to report their census, balance sheet, income statement, expenses, cash forecast, budget, expenses, or receivables in a predetermined format. The regulatory agency determines the precise format by which such data are reported. The purpose of this request is to facilitate accumulation, analysis, and comparison of performance data over all organizations. The end results of this analysis are often the setting of reimbursement rates or the determination of allowable costs. Such activities are obviously facilitated where information has been provided to the regulatory agency or third party payer in a standardized format in advance.

Third parties are continually interested in the expenditure trends by the health facilities they reimburse. Consequently they need precise data to make decisions on their reimbursement policies and to address equity of payment to any single health care organization. As a result, more states have adopted uniform reporting to remove the discrepancies in how financial data are reported. However, uniform reporting also has its analog at the organization level. The decision support system should process reports on a periodic basis to facilitate decision making and planning. These reports also fall into the category of uniform reporting.

Using Management Reports

Beyond the basic reports of the balance sheet, income statement, and statement of changes in financial position, it is appropriate for nursing administrators and other health care managers to employ certain supplemental reports in controlling operations.[1] This fact is particularly relevant to health care organizations that confront pluralistic funding sources and offer a diverse set of services or products. Furthermore, the growth of computerized decision support or management information systems has opened possibilities for more reports than ever before possible.[2,3] In fact, the availability of these systems and their output is something of a problem if discretion is not used in selecting which reports are required. Without such control there is a potential for a profusion of reports that confuse rather than clarify management decisions. For these reasons, nursing administrators must be very careful in determining what reports they need to direct their operations.

It is important to recognize that not every management situation requires a complex computerized information system or set of reports. There is a convincing argument that many situations can even be handled quite adequately without the computer-generated reports. This is particularly true for the smaller health care facility or program without the resources to tap into a sophisticated data management system. In those situations it is appropriate to ascertain whether data can be accurately accumulated on a consistent basis by manual means. A problem results when the data can be easily accessed but there are pressures that prevent consistent implementation of the system.

With these considerations in mind, it is still essential for nurse administrators and other health care managers to carefully select the strategy that accomplishes their goals best. Other than the performance reports discussed above, it may be necessary for managers to acquire report data that allow them to make decisions on current operations. Such a portfolio of reports must include at least two items—a report on current operating performance and a report on statistical performance.

Table 2–9 depicts a report on operating performance that conveys the general format that may be useful in managing current operations. Any health care manager must be alert to current trends in patient revenues. Of concern is the direction of each specific payer in terms of levels of revenues. Questions are constantly at issue in examining these data: Have there been major shifts from one payer to another in terms of revenues at the inpatient and outpatient levels? What do these shifts imply for the program services offered? How has the profile of patients changed as a result of the changes in payer mix? What sorts of staffing or resource investment decisions will have to be made to account for the changing payer mix? This sort of questioning and hypothesizing is most relevant to management reports. It is at this level that the regeneration of the organization begins to take place as it strives to remain competitive and cognizant of its environment.

Table 2–9 Report on Operating Performance

	Current Month			Year-to-Date		
	Actual	Budgeted	Variance	Actual	Budgeted	Variance
Patient Revenues						
Inpatient Total						
Medicare						
Medicaid						
Blue Cross						
Self-Pay						
Other Carriers						
Outpatient Total						
Medicare						
Medicaid						
Blue Cross						
Self-Pay						
Other Carriers						
Gross Patient Revenues						
Allowances and Uncollectibles						
Contractual Allowances Total						
Medicare						
Medicaid						
Blue Cross						
Other Contractual						
Uncollectible Accounts						
(Bad Debt)						
Net Patient Revenue						
Other Revenue						
Total Net Revenue						
Expenses						
Salaries and Wages						
(by job category)						
Benefits						
Contractual Personnel Costs						
Depreciation						
Maintenance						
Interest						
Property Taxes						
Other Expenses						
Net Income						

Beyond patient revenues, a nursing administrator may find it useful to periodically assess other performance areas shown in Table 2–9. Certainly relevant in this regard are the areas of expenses and net performance (e.g., income and revenue). The financially oriented manager needs to know where expenses are being incurred at varying levels compared with those expenses forecasted. Awareness establishes a basis for action.

Table 2–10 depicts another useful management report. Statistical performance related to utilization is vital to any health care organization.[4] Managers must determine what is occurring in terms of patient use. Such a report can be constructed for overall operations and clinic operations as shown in Table 2–10. Alternatively, such a report can concentrate on only one aspect of an organization's performance.

The nurse administrator should recognize that there is no ultimate set of operations or utilization reports. The needs of the organization or department must determine which reports are eventually created. Once the reports have been created, it is then the responsibility of the nurse administrator to put the reports into action. Here is where most managers fail miserably. A report is a guide to planning and decision making. It should facilitate decisions, not take them from managers. At the same time it is vital that managers not adopt a position that reports are a waste of time—that the manager already knows the trends. Take time to scrutinize reports because they help take the pulse of an organization or program. Once that pulse has been determined, the reports may then provide the rationale for selecting among various program or strategy alternatives.

Table 2–10 Report on Statistical Performance

Overall Operations
1. Total Patient Days
2. Average Daily Census
3. Occupancy
4. Average Length of Stay
5. Admissions
6. Discharges
7. Patient Days by Payer
   Medicare
   Medicaid
   Blue Cross
   Commercial Insurance
   Self-Pay
   Other
8. Trends in Twenty Most Profitable DRGs
9. Trends in Twenty Most Costly DRGs

Clinic Operations
1. Total Encounters
2. Encounters by Type of Service
3. Encounters per FTE Staff
4. Encounters by Payer

PROSPECTIVE PAYMENT AND FINANCIAL REPORTS

The admonitions that nurse administrators and other health care managers should carefully contemplate the types of reports they request, and the extent to which they actually use the reports, are especially important in view of prospective payment. There is certainly little doubt that the need for careful financial management of health care organizations has taken a quantum leap with the introduction of prospective payment. Such payment systems have increased the necessity for deliberate and accurate analysis of performance. Reports on cost performance within specific diagnosis groups is a perfect illustration of new reports that are receiving close scrutiny by many health care managers.

These trends toward prospective payment and increased analytical management are likely to continue in the future. The buffers of slack resources and generous reimbursement have rapidly disappeared in the health care field. The prognosis is for such pressures to continue in the future. Consequently nurse administrators must recognize that they can only help their departments, programs, work units, and organizations overcome these pressures when they have accurate information for making decisions and plans.

NOTES

1. Ralph B. Tower, "Analyzing Accounting Reports," *Nursing Management* 13 (September 1982): 12–16.
2. George Coulter, "CFO's Role Changes in Systems Planning and Operations," *Healthcare Financial Management* 40 (February 1986): 54–55.
3. Gordon A. King, "Choosing and Using Electronic Spreadsheets: The Financial Manager's New Best Friend," *Healthcare Financial Management* 39 (January 1985): 54–60.
4. James C. Rickard, "Making It Easier for the Financial Manager," *Healthcare Financial Management* 37 (June 1983): 32, 36.

Chapter 3

Assessing Financial Performance

With the trend toward multi-institutional health care organizations and rising corporate involvement in the health field, it is becoming increasingly important to be able to compare financial performance over a given fiscal period. The ability to compare and contrast financial performance from one organization to the next, or to assess performance over several years, may provide some indication of the effectiveness of managerial action or the appropriateness of merger. Yet such analysis is difficult to undertake. There is a problem of a lack of comparability in the information presented in financial statements. Consequently it is difficult to know whether a correct comparison is being made. Added to this problem is the issue of adjusting for the size of one health care organization versus another. Without standards that adjust for factors such as magnitude of revenues, expenses, capitalization, fixed assets, or current obligations, any comparison is tenuous at best.

The problem of comparing the performance of one health care organization with another is compounded because standards are lacking and health care organizations are very dynamic. For example, how can it be ascertained that the financial performance of one hospital is better than another? Simply looking at liquidity and net revenues would not truly provide a fair basis of comparison. Perhaps one of the hospitals has recently divested current assets (e.g., an inventory of special equipment) in order to allocate the liquidity toward operating funds. This divestment would have the effect of raising total operating funds, assuming that the inventory was sold at a profitable level. This example indicates these important concepts:

- Financial performance must be assessed through a comprehensive set of measures.
- Valid assessments of performance should incorporate more than one fiscal period.

- An evaluation of performance is most useful when there is a comparison to similar organizations within the health care field.

As with most forms of evaluation, the assessment of financial performance can be conducted in many ways. However, there are some commonly accepted principles that can guide such analyses.

Nurse administrators should attempt to understand the relevance of assessing the financial performance of an organization. Whether for-profit or nonprofit, a health care organization must attain financial solvency and provide a good return on r⁻ ᵒurces if it expects to survive over the long run.[1] Even if it is able to perform adequately in attaining patient care goals and financial goals, there is always the question of whether performance could have been improved. Unfortunately many health care managers become complacent in terms of driving their organizations toward better performance.

The chief financial officer is responsible for maintaining control over financial operations, but the responsibility for financial operations does not stop there. There must be some level of internal motivation among management staff that enables the organization to repeatedly question how it can perform better. This is the duty of the chief financial officer in terms of total financial performance, but it is also the responsibility of nurse administrators in terms of striving toward better financially oriented performance within their departments, programs, or work units. The accumulation of these efforts eventually should result in improved overall performance.

If nurse administrators do not have the skill to assess the financial well-being of their departments or work units, then they probably have a limited basis for assessing the performance of the total organization. Only by developing a solid background in assessing overall performance, including financial operations, can a nurse administrator begin to understand the critical factors that affect nursing's contribution to costs and revenue. Once that knowledge of financial effectiveness is attained, it is easier to communicate with other managers in the organization. An analytical framework exists for adjusting the operations of the nursing unit in order to achieve better performance both within the unit and within the organization.

ASSESSMENT TOOLS

When it comes to assessing financial performance, there are innumerable methodologies and tools available to the financially knowledgeable manager. The foundation for assessment begins with basic statistics on operations—particularly statistics surrounding financial operations. As is common for most for-profit, nonprofit, and government organizations, the basic information needed to make the assessments is reported in financial statements. The ability to read financial statements is probably most critical to ensuing analysis.[2] The financial statements present descriptive data on operations. The balance sheet, statement of revenues and expenses, and statement of changes in financial position are prevalent methods for reporting data from which additional analysis can commence.

Sophisticated financial analysis must rely on the information that is presented in basic financial reports. A critical premise is that the data are accurate. This may be an erroneous assumption. Even with the use of accounting experts to certify data, usually a high degree of subjectivity enters into the reporting of financial data. This is true for most organizations that have complex operations and diverse sources of funds. However, there is little that an analyst can do to improve the data. This point is made in order to alert nurse administrators to a key premise underlying the fundamental analysis of financial data. There are inherent inconsistencies in the data that may confound even the most precise efforts at analysis. Comparisons of performance, therefore, may be based on incorrect assumptions.

In all practicality, these problems with the accuracy of reported financial data are seldom completely resolved. Therefore performance assessment appears to be more an art than a science. Nonetheless, nurse administrators should understand financial analysis to the fullest extent possible. This understanding would help them to correctly interpret reports on financial performance and to temper their comparisons, decisions, conclusions, and forecasts when using the data. As greater familiarity with the reports and the sources of data is developed, it will be easier to understand and interpret the inherent limitations. The purpose is to reach an accurate interpretation of the performance for nursing services.

Beyond the standard financial reports, there are several methods that can be used to analyze the data contained in the reports. The most prevalent method for assessing financial performance beyond merely reading standardized reports is to use ratios, indices, or indicators constructed from report data. Financial ratios are a useful convention to assess a given organization's performance or to compare the performance of that organization with others of a similar type.

Above all, ratios provide a logical methodology. Remember that the data in financial statements for even a small hospital or nursing home are numerous and complex. It would be easy to become confused by these data or to focus on one aspect of performance to the exclusion of other areas in view of the overwhelming amount. Much more important than the possibility of overlooking an aspect of financial performance is the problem of not recognizing the dynamic interrelationships among variables.

For example, what happens to the statement of revenues and expenses when a health maintenance organization secures more long-term debt in order to finance a clinic? What happens to the balance sheet and income statement when a nursing home suddenly reduces its accounts receivable? These are only a few of the questions that in turn generate further questions on the financial performance of an organization. If a convenient mechanism is not available for portraying changes in these variables, excessive time would be wasted in tracing the impact from financial report to financial report. Hence the probability of error would increase.

A resolution to this dilemma can be achieved by calculating standardized ratios. These ratios can be quickly determined and therefore they facilitate an understanding of overall financial performance and of management effectiveness for a health care organization. Financial analysts have defined an extensive set of ratios that are useful for analyzing not only the performance of a given organization but also an entire industry of organizations. These ratios are particularly useful in plotting changes in financial performance from one fiscal period to the next. They are a visual aid to the analysis of financial outcomes. Furthermore, these ratios provide a useful basis for comparison when analyzing the financial performance of one organization compared with others in the same industry.

Financial managers typically use ratio analysis to identify problems in profitability, activity, or capitalization of an organization. As such, the ratios help them pinpoint causal relationships that are negatively affecting performance. Once alerted to these problems, it is possible to create more satisfactory solutions in a more timely fashion. This point is often overlooked because financial ratios are used predominantly by individuals, agencies, and groups outside the organization's boundary. Ratio analysis is used by investors, brokerage firms, lenders, security analysts, or other parties who want to compare financial performance among organizations or assess the financial health of an organization. Nonetheless, ratio analysis should be equally prevalent in managing the overall operations of a given health care organization.

From one perspective, ratio analysis is advocated as an essential management tool.[3] Not only does ratio analysis provide managers with standardized methods for comparing performance, it also helps to identify weaknesses in financial performance. Once the health care manager is aware of these inherent problems, it is possible to create plans that resolve the problems. In general, ratio analysis receives such favorable support because it represents the injection of rigorous business practices into the financial management of health care organizations. The result is more analytical planning and decision making, combined with less subjectivity in managing financial issues.

Another view of financial ratios suggests much greater caution in their use and interpretation.[4,5] According to this perspective, financial ratios are easily influenced by inflation, trends that may be the result of spurious causes, and the lack of comparability among organizations. Therefore health care managers should be encouraged not to overrely on the ratios and their implications. By relying too extensively on ratios, the manager may actually be misinterpreting the performance of an organization. Hidden facts, forces, and trends may make the ratios appear better (or worse) than performance actually is, all things considered. The best response for nurse administrators or other health care managers interested in financial ratios is to use ratios as an important starting point for further analysis.

Confirm the implications suggested by ratios. Never assume that ratios present a final, accurate profile.

RATIO ANALYSIS

There are four main categories of ratios used by managers and analysts to assess financial performance:

1. Liquidity ratios indicate the extent to which short-run obligations can be met.
2. Profitability ratios define the extent of net revenue and usually compare it with a given level of equity.
3. Activity ratios measure the efficiency of an organization in using its assets.
4. Leverage ratios describe the amount of debt relative to equity.

Not all categories of ratios are used equally among managers and analysts. The key criterion in determining their use is the goal of the analysis in the first place. Profitability and activity ratios are good indicators of current operations. Liquidity ratios define the amount of current risk in meeting obligations. The leverage ratios capture the long-run perspective of the firm in the sense of its ability to regenerate its capital and to plan for judicious growth of the asset base.

Beyond the four categories mentioned above, organizations often use additional ratios that are germane to their particular industry. This is precisely the case for the health care field. Third party reimbursement makes imperative the use of supplemental ratios that are not normally found in business organizations. There is a significant difference in how equity is treated in health care organizations as compared with business corporations. The need to separate funds into restricted and unrestricted fund balances is very important. Fund accounting is a major consideration given the nonprofit nature of the health care industry.[6] These distinctive aspects of health care organizations can be easily incorporated through supplemental ratios.

Financial ratios can best be conveyed and explained by examining how they are constructed from balance sheets and income statements. In facilitating this analysis, we will consider the abbreviated case of a 100-bed nonprofit hospital located in the Midwest. Sierra Hospital's balance sheet is shown in Table 3–1.

The balance sheet indicates that Sierra Hospital in its last fiscal period had total current liabilities of $1,137,000 and total long-run liabilities of $4,412,000. The fund balance was $7,564,000. These liabilities are balanced against $9,098,000 in existing plant and equipment as well as a reserve fund for new plant construction. The hospital has $4,015,000 in current assets.

Table 3–1 Balance Sheet for Sierra Hospital

Current Assets		
Cash	$	194,000
Marketable Securities		78,000
Accounts Receivable		2,743,000
Inventory		301,000
Miscellaneous Current Assets		699,000
Total Current Assets		4,015,000
Fixed Assets		
Plant		6,711,000
Equipment		1,871,000
Plant Fund		516,000
Total Fixed Assets		9,098,000
Total Assets		$13,113,000
Current Liabilities		
Accounts Payable	$	984,000
Salaries Payable		153,000
Total Current Liabilities		1,137,000
Long-Term Liabilities		
Mortgage Bonds		2,733,000
Other Long-Term Debt		1,679,000
Fund Balance		7,564,000
Total Long-Term Liabilities and Equity		11,976,000
Total Liabilities		$13,113,000

The income statement or statement of revenue and expenses for Sierra Hospital is shown in Table 3–2. This financial report suggests that the last fiscal period was very lucrative for the hospital. Net income was $2,695,000 on the basis of $10,097,000 in total operating revenue after discounts and allowances. Operating expenses totaled $8,345,000. The operating margin was supplemented by $943,000 in other revenue. Overall, the income statement suggests that Sierra Hospital is in a good position as far as its use of its assets.

The question that must be answered is: how well has Sierra Hospital been performing? One method for answering this question would be to go through each item listed on the balance sheet and income statement and try to explain how it relates to others. Since there are 19 entries on the balance sheet and 16 entries on the income statement, such an approach would be laborious, duplicative, and therefore might overlook some key information or trends relevant to the decision maker. Note that even with the simple financial statements depicted in Tables 3–1 and 3–2, the amount of information is overwhelming. This is where financial

Table 3–2 Income Statement for Sierra Hospital

Patient Revenues	$10,274,000
Less: Discounts and Allowances for Bad Debts	511,000
	9,763,000
Other Sources of Revenue	334,000
Total Operating Revenue	10,097,000
Operating Expenses	
Nursing Care	3,125,000
General and Administrative	329,000
Clinical Fees	1,347,000
Dietary	1,573,000
Housekeeping	1,700,000
Depreciation	196,000
Interest	75,000
	8,345,000
Operating Income	1,752,000
Nonoperating Revenue	943,000
Net Income	$ 2,695,000

ratios are especially beneficial. However, contemplate how difficult such comparisons would be in the event of a complex balance sheet and income statement for a 300-bed hospital. The amount of information is excessive and thereby limits the precision of the analysis.

In view of the preceding thoughts, nurse administrators should recognize the fundamental advantages of financial ratios. At this point it is appropriate to discuss each category of ratios and define the specific ratios that compose these main categories. Then the ratios will be applied to Sierra Hospital in order to illustrate how they can be computed from the information supplied in the financial statements.

Liquidity Ratios

Liquidity ratios measure the extent to which short-run obligations can be met by the organization.[7] The main resources to be used in meeting these obligations are current assets that are highly liquid. In this sense, it is possible that a health care facility may be low on actual cash, but high on accounts receivable. Since receivables will shortly be transformed into cash or can be used as collateral for borrowing, they are also a useful standard for measuring liquidity. However, if a firm is not able to meet its current obligations by liquidating assets, then its long-run prognosis is poor. Liquidity must be interpreted in relation to all aspects of financial performance.

Current Ratio

The current ratio is calculated in the following manner:

$$\text{Current Ratio (CR)} = \frac{\text{Current Assets}}{\text{Current Liabilities}}$$

$$\text{Sierra Hospital CR} = \frac{\$4,015,000}{\$1,137,000} = 3.53$$

According to this ratio, Sierra Hospital has almost three times more current assets compared with current liabilities. It is in a good financial position because it could incur substantially more current obligations or debt (i.e., \$4,015,000 − \$1,137,000 = \$2,878,000) before it would be unable to pay off these bills. Note that simply because the current ratio is high (i.e., indicates good ability to pay current debts) does not imply that Sierra Hospital is maintaining a policy of good financial management. In fact just the opposite may be true. When current assets become too high there is the implication that the earning power of assets has diminished. Specifically, some of the current assets could be invested in higher interest-bearing accounts or in long-term ventures. Sierra Hospital's cash position (i.e., \$194,000) appears to be relatively high.

It is important to observe the duality conveyed by the ratio. A low current ratio may not imply that current assets are too low; current liabilities may be too high. This could imply that health care managers need to concentrate more on containing costs. Perhaps an excessive amount of spending has occurred just before the close of the fiscal period. As a result, the current ratio in the ensuing period would be lower.

Acid Test Ratio

The acid test or so-called quick ratio is calculated as follows:

$$\text{Acid Test Ratio (ATR)} = \frac{\text{Current Assets} - \text{Inventory}}{\text{Current Liabilities}}$$

$$\text{Sierra Hospital ATR} = \frac{\$4,015,000 - \$301,000}{\$1,137,000} = 3.27$$

The acid test ratio adjusts current assets for the existing volume of inventory. The rationale for this adjustment relates to the nature of most corporate inventories. Inventory is an excellent marketable commodity. However, inventory is not a negotiable instrument and therefore it has value primarily when there is market demand. The market demand for a product can vary, and in some instances approaches the condition of being like cash (i.e., goods are sold just as soon as they are made available to customers). In other cases, inventory may be held for months until it is converted into cash. For most health care organizations, inventory is highly perishable because it consists of pharmaceuticals or food supplies. Nonetheless the level of inventory for a given hospital, clinic, or nursing home is much less than for business corporations because the health care organization produces services rather than goods.

Note that the acid test ratio for Sierra Hospital is only marginally influenced by the deletion of inventory. The same dynamic relationship among variables pertains to the acid test ratio as the current ratio. In other words, the specific causal factor for a low or high value is determined by either the liabilities or the assets. By calculating the acid test ratio, the manager can be alerted to a financial condition that would have gone unnoted had the calculation never been made.

Days in Accounts Receivable

Hospitals and other health care organizations are unlike typical business enterprises.[8] They receive substantial funding from third party payers over whom they have little control. Transactions are seldom cash- or credit-based. Usually complex billing must be undertaken in order to recover revenue for a transaction. These facts make it important for every health care organization to monitor the number of days that pass before bills are paid by third party payers and other payers in the health system. Money has true value, and the longer bills are not paid by customers (i.e., by their sources of insurance) the more likely the bills are to remain unpaid, and the less efficient is the management of current operations (because less interest can be earned on the dollars held in accounts receivable).

The days in accounts receivable is calculated as:

$$\text{Days in Accounts Receivable (DAR)} = \frac{\text{Net Accounts Receivable} \times 365}{\text{Net Operating Revenue}}$$

$$\text{Sierra Hospital DAR} = \frac{(\$2,743,000) \times 365}{\$9,763,000} = 102.5$$

The days in accounts receivable indicates the length of time it takes to collect on charges. When there is a high value for this ratio the implication is that money that could otherwise be invested is being held in a noncash form by accounts receivable—usually third party payers. Like any business, a health care organization has bills to pay. Unless it receives payment for expenses incurred in delivering services it will go bankrupt. Hospitals and other health care organizations are, after all, not banking institutions. They are not in the money lending business, hence they should not operate like a bank when it comes to receivables. Unfortunately this is more the case than an exception to the rule.

When the days in accounts receivable is excessively high, the health care organization has ample reasons to suspect that management action is needed. Attention can be focused on many aspects of collections and current operations. It may be judicious to evaluate the collections system—particular attention should focus on the billing system and medical records. Does medical records submit documentation early enough that a bill avoids delinquency prior to leaving the health care organization? There is sufficient reason to concentrate on billing in view of the tightening controls over prospective payments. Billing is essential to the accounts receivable area and should receive appropriate attention from management.

Another consideration in a high accounts receivable figure is the possibility that the health care organization is carrying many old accounts that have a limited probability of being paid. A high percentage of late accounts will never be collected and should be written off the books as bad debts. Added effort should then be made at the time of admission to prevent similar uncollectible accounts from occurring in the future. This might require more extensive patient counseling or creation of ingenious payment plans that facilitate rather than intimidate marginal but willing patients.

In the case of Sierra Hospital, the days in accounts receivable figure is 102.5 days. This is generally quite high because it implies that it takes over three months to collect on any account. In other words, some accounts are taking even longer than three months to collect. Action is vitally needed to prevent this figure from rising any higher because Sierra Hospital is actually losing income in the form of interest. It is possible, however, that the fiscal year ends at a time when seasonality has substantial influence over the ratio. Although this argument diminishes when assessing financial performance from year to year (because each year experiences the same seasonality), there is justification for analysis that would focus on the direct causes of the anomaly. Several alternative hypotheses should be considered as to why the ratio is beyond acceptable standards.

Average Payment Period

The reciprocal of the days in accounts receivable is the average payment period. This ratio measures the length of time in days that it takes a health care organization to pay its own debts:

$$\text{Average Payment Period (APP)} = \frac{\text{Current Liabilities} \times 365}{\text{Total Operating Expenses} - \text{Depreciation}}$$

$$\text{Sierra Hospital APP} = \frac{\$1,137,000 \times 365}{\$8,345,000 - \$196,000} = 50.9$$

The average payment period for Sierra Hospital is 50.9 days. This figure suggests that it takes Sierra Hospital roughly one-half the time to pay its own bills that it takes for other entities to pay the receivables owed to Sierra Hospital.

In terms of liquidity, the average payment period provides insight into the ability of an organization to pay its bills. The longer that is required to pay these bills, the more likely that at least one of two things has gone wrong: either (1) there are too many current liabilities or (2) total operating expenses and depreciation are too high. Note that in the case of total operating expenses, an adjustment is made in subtracting out depreciation because depreciation is a noncash expense. There is no direct outlay of funds, hence there is no actual bill to pay.

Days Cash On Hand

Perhaps the ultimate measure of liquidity is the average number of days of cash on hand:

$$\frac{\text{Average Days}}{\text{Cash on Hand (DCH)}} = \frac{(\text{Marketable Securities} + \text{Cash}) \times 365}{\text{Total Operating Expense} - \text{Depreciation Expense}}$$

$$\text{Sierra Hospital DCH} = \frac{(\$78,000 + \$194,000) \times 365}{\$8,345,000 - \$196,000} = 12.2$$

The days cash on hand ratio assesses the liquidity of the health care organization from the perspective of cash and marketable securities. It provides a good measure of the extent to which available cash or liquid securities could be used to pay daily expenses. Although a high figure implies much cash and hence low risk, questions must be raised about whether such cash is excessive. Too much cash and marketable securities implies that management has not been taking advantage of opportunities to invest in securities, ventures, and assets that could produce a higher return.

In the case of Sierra Hospital the number of days cash on hand (DCH) ratio suggests that the hospital can adequately pay for all daily bills for up to twelve days before its cash reserves run out. This assumes that there will be no other cash flowing into the organization during that time. This, of course, is not often found in reality. Generally a health care organization will maintain a daily flow of revenue. This is implied in the receivables figure. While not all of the receivables will be spread out evenly each day, operational cash flow does limit the immediate threat of suddenly being unable to pay certain bills.

The question is whether Sierra Hospital's days cash on hand ratio is too low. If anything, this ratio appears to be too high. Unless the hospital is planning for a major expenditure in the near future, $194,000 is generally a large amount of cash to have immediately available for an organization with $10,274,000 in patient revenues. This ratio could easily be cut in half and still the degree of risk would be low. Alternatively, it is possible to view operating expenses as low. This may be due to a conscientious cost control program that has effectively lowered the ratio. In this regard the effectiveness of lowering costs is reaped in terms of more cash and lower expenses.

Profitability Ratios

The concept of return on investment will become increasingly dominant in the health care field in the future.[9] Tightening restraints on third party payments make it imperative that health care organizations obtain the most efficient performance in order to meet financial solvency goals.[10] Meanwhile, the expanding corporate orientation of the health industry will gradually raise the preeminence of the profit goal. Investor-owned health care corporations will produce a powerful influence over the managerial outlook in the future. Unless sufficient profits are made, capital will leave the industry. From the single institution's perspective, it must be able to derive profitability in order to meet corporate goals and to fulfill its own quality and profitability goals.

In view of the growing interest in the profitability of health care organizations, it is essential that a convenient framework be established to identify profitable operations. This framework should be capable of identifying health care organizations that have attained a satisfactory level of profit on services rendered. This idea applies to a lesser extent in the case of nonprofit institutions, but there still is a critical demand for nonprofit organizations to act as good stewards of their resources.[11] In essence they too must achieve profitability if they expect to survive over the long run. The profitability ratios represent an effective device for assessing the profitability of health care organizations.

Return on Equity (Fund Balance)

Foremost in the minds of investors is the extent of return on equity invested in an organization. This key ratio is calculated in the following fashion:

$$\text{Return on Equity (ROE)} = \frac{\text{Net Income}}{\text{Fund Balance}}$$

$$\text{Sierra Hospital ROE} = \frac{\$2,695,000}{\$7,564,000} = .36$$

As this ratio suggests, the primary interest of health care managers is to maximize the amount of net income earned relative to total equity (or fund balance). As the organization becomes more highly capitalized (i.e., investors have put more capital into the organization), the ability to derive profits should increase, otherwise the capital should not be invested in the first place. The concern of investors is to see their investment make money; the concern of managers is to make certain that it does. Thus, the goal of investing capital in enterprises that make certain goods and services is to obtain a financial return on that investment.

There are essentially two directions in which the return on equity ratio can vary. If the fund balance is low—indicating little investment on the part of the owners—then net income is in effect supported. Less overall income is needed to produce a good return on a small capital base. Similarly, a high magnitude of net income will compensate for a large fund balance. The ability to earn net income will positively influence the return on equity ratio. By achieving efficiency with invested capital, the manager is able to derive high profits from a limited capital investment.

In the case of Sierra Hospital, the return on equity ratio is .36 or a 36 percent return on investment for the past fiscal year. For virtually any investment, this figure is exemplary. For a health care organization it is more than exceptional. What factors have contributed to this level of performance? Examining the income statement in Table 3–2, we see that several factors have contributed to the performance:

- Patient revenues are high, yet there is a low proportion of discounts and allowances for bad debts.
- Other sources of revenue have almost balanced the bad debt level.
- Operating expenses are low relative to patient revenues.
- Nonoperating revenue is very high given the level of patient revenues.

From a complete perspective, it is probable that low costs represent the single most important factor in the high net income.

Table 3–1, the balance sheet for Sierra Hospital, also provides some evidence about the performance of the return on equity. The fund balance figure is very low given the high amount of net income earned. It appears that the resources that have been invested are being used very effectively in terms of overall financial operations.

Return on Total Assets

The return on total assets ratio represents the return earned by a health care organization for all investors including lenders. Remember that any individual or party that lends money to an organization is in essence investing in the organization. In the case of Sierra Hospital these investments are then translated into fixed and current assets. Sierra Hospital is maintaining $4,015,000 of current assets and $9,098,000 of fixed assets. Therefore it is appropriate to look at the return on these assets, since they represent the current and future productivity of the hospital. While the return on equity ratio provides insight into the actual amount of resources owned, the return on total assets ratio provides an analysis of how the total available resources are earning income.

The return on total assets ratio is calculated as:

$$\text{Return on Total Assets (ROA)} = \frac{\text{Net Income}}{\text{Total Assets}}$$

$$\text{Sierra Hospital ROA} = \frac{\$2,695,000}{\$13,113,000} = .21$$

Once again the ratio is exceptionally high. This result suggests that Sierra Hospital is using all of its current and fixed assets at an exceptional level of performance.

Operating Margin

Business organizations attempt to assess the respective percentage of sales that eventually will result in profits. Although health care organizations do not make sales in the strict sense of the word, they do acquire revenues in compensation for their charges. Hence they are interested in ascertaining their net operating margin on total patient revenues:

$$\text{Operating Margin (OM)} = \frac{\text{Operating Income}}{\text{Total Operating Revenue}}$$

$$\text{Sierra Hospital OM} = \frac{\$1,752,000}{\$10,097,000} = .17$$

Note that nonoperating revenues have been omitted from the calculation of this ratio. This is the result of determining the profitability of patient revenues before adding in nonoperating revenues. The operating margin provides a measure of the effectiveness or productivity of patient care services in providing net income to the health care organization. In the case of Sierra Hospital, the operating margin is .17, which suggests that 17 percent of all operating revenues—patient revenues (less discounts and allowances) and related service revenues—eventually end up as net income. This is excellent performance.

Nonoperating Revenue Ratio

Health care organizations are unique when compared with business organizations in that they have supplemental sources of income derived from endowments, gift shops, parking, management fees, and other nonpatient care revenues. From a financial solvency perspective, a high level of nonoperating revenue is positive because it implies that there are other sources of income beyond just patient care that supplement overall operations. If these revenues are especially profitable, then there are more resources to cover the costs of inpatient services. However, excessive nonpatient care revenues can have a negative influence if a high level of these revenues is being derived at the expense of patient care. In such a situation, the attention of managers may have focused extensively on raising the nonpatient care revenues. Attention to cost control or patient marketing strategies may have been minimized. These latter strategies could be used to improve operating revenues.

This argument is not insignificant given changes in the health care field. Diversification is an increasingly prevalent phenomenon among health care organizations. Admittedly, diversification usually results in major enterprises related to patient care, which implies that revenues will be categorized under operating revenues. In other cases a separate organizational entity is established where the health care organization functions as a holding company. The point is that diversification does not guarantee that new revenues will necessarily be accounted for as operating revenues. However, in hospitals that limit their diversification activities, it is possible to raise nonoperating income.

For example, a hospital might undertake diversification into prenatal parent education and wellness programs. Both could easily be classified as nonpatient care services, and as a result, it is likely that they will be incorporated into the nonoperating revenue category. Since the services are not patient care oriented on either an outpatient or inpatient basis, it is likely that they will not be viewed as mainline patient care services. Diversification, therefore, expands the base of nonoperating revenue.

The nonoperating revenue ratio is calculated as:

$$\text{Nonoperating Revenue Ratio (NOR)} = \frac{\text{Nonoperating Revenue}}{\text{Net Income}}$$

$$\text{Sierra Hospital NOR} = \frac{\$943,000}{\$2,695,000} = .35$$

Sierra Hospital has a high level of nonoperating revenue relative to net income. This implies that either the level of nonoperating revenue is very high or operating income is low. The income statement for Sierra Hospital suggests it is more likely that nonoperating revenue is high. The operating income is very good in view of the expenses to revenues for patient care. Therefore it appears that Sierra Hospital has been successful in deriving revenues beyond patient care services.

Discounts and Allowances Ratio

A ratio with growing importance to health care managers is the extent of discounts and allowances. This ratio conveys the level of bad debts, contractual allowances, charity care, and any other price reductions given to patients. Since hospitals are experiencing tighter constraints on their revenue, a high ratio for discounts and allowances must cause alarm. It implies that deserved revenue is not being acquired. It implies that patients who can pay are actually not paying (e.g., bad debts). It implies that a large portion of the patient population will not pay because they lack the capability (i.e., charity care). With the growing restrictions on third party payment, it will become increasingly more difficult for hospitals to justify these nonpaying patients.

The discounts and allowances ratio is calculated in the following manner:

$$\text{Discounts and Allowances (DA)} = \frac{\text{Discounts, Allowances, and Uncollectibles}}{\text{Patient Revenue}}$$

$$\text{Sierra Hospital DA} = \frac{\$511,000}{\$10,097,000} = .05$$

Sierra Hospital has a discounts and allowances ratio of .05. This means that approximately five percent of all patient revenue is never actually collected due to bad debts, charity care, or contractual allowances. Although this figure is not excessive compared with other hospitals, or even with business organizations and their trade discounts, the matter is really a relative issue. If health care organizations continue to experience restraints on revenue, then the proportion of free care and other allowances becomes very important in determining financial solvency. It is likely that the discounts and allowances ratio will receive more attention by health care financial officers in the near future.

Activity Ratios

The purpose of activity ratios is to provide financial officers with an understanding of how assets contribute to total operating revenue. As such, activity ratios indicate how well assets are managed. Do they work hard in order to generate revenues, or are they managed in a less concentrated effort to derive patient care revenues? From the health care manager's view, the activity ratios are important in determining whether he/she is doing a good job of stewardship over the assets.

When an activity ratio is low, there is an implication that the assets should be reorganized to produce more. Counterbalancing this claim is the problem of the age of the assets. Even though the value of assets may be very high, there is a possibility that they have lost their flexibility for generating patient revenues.

An additional useful aspect of activity ratios is the ability to assess overinvestment in either current or fixed assets. For a health care organization, an excessive investment in current assets may mean that productivity is being lost because current assets generally are highly liquid and do not relate to patient care. Unlike business corporations, a health care organization is less concerned with inventory because it produces services rather than goods. Thus, the most likely problem is remaining too liquid and therefore nonproductive in terms of current assets. There is also a danger in being overinvested in fixed assets from the perspective of not being able to meet current obligations. It usually takes excessive time to divest the fixed assets to obtain liquidity. Generally the approach is to retain the fixed assets and borrow the needed funds. This cost of short-term capital is usually more expensive than the firm's cost of capital, and hence a strategy to be avoided.

Total Asset Turnover

The total asset turnover ratio calculates the extent to which all assets are being used effectively to generate operating revenues:

$$\text{Total Asset Turnover (TAT)} = \frac{\text{Total Operating Revenue}}{\text{Total Assets}}$$

$$\text{Sierra Hospital TAT} = \frac{\$10,097,000}{\$13,113,000} = .77$$

The relationship between the two variables—revenue and assets—is like many other ratios examined to this point. If total assets are low, and they are being used effectively, then the net effect is to produce a high amount of total operating revenues and hence a high ratio. If the assets are not productive then the total asset turnover ratio will be low because few revenues are being created through the assets.

It must be remembered that a high proportion of assets within any health care organization is devoted to services that generate total revenues. When these services are not being managed efficiently there can be a deleterious effect on resulting revenues. It is not the assets themselves that are productive in the case of the hospital, but rather the services that are housed within the assets or that use the assets. This is an important distinction that should be remembered when we assess any activity ratio and particularly total asset turnover.

Sierra Hospital's total asset turnover ratio is .77, which is somewhat below normal for hospitals. Compared with corporations, this figure is well below published norms. The implication is that Sierra Hospital is not being very efficient in managing its total investment. However, it is critical to consider the nature of health care services. The assets are not mass producing specific goods but rather establishing a setting for services. Also of consideration is the fact that the assets themselves may be new and not yet depreciated. In this case, the facilities at Sierra Hospital may not be managed very efficiently in terms of overall operations. Alternatively, it can be argued that Sierra Hospital has an extensively depreciated asset base that is losing its productive capacity.

Current Asset Turnover

The current asset turnover ratio measures the efficiency of current assets to generate revenues:

$$\text{Current Asset Turnover (CAT)} = \frac{\text{Total Operating Revenue}}{\text{Current Assets}}$$

$$\text{Sierra Hospital CAT} = \frac{\$10,097,000}{\$\ 4,015,000} = 2.15$$

This ratio must be used with some caution in health care organizations because of the nature of the industry. Current assets for most health care institutions include two important items—accounts receivable and inventory. Accounts receivable is by far the more important concern. Since receivables constitute a high percentage of current assets, the current asset turnover ratio indirectly is a comment on receivables. Are receivables related to total operating revenue? Clearly the higher the amount of revenue generated, the larger will be the receivables. In a similar vein, inventory is related to total operating revenue in the sense that more revenue implies the delivery of more services and hence the need for a higher base of inventory.

The current asset turnover ratio is important in conveying the ability of a health care organization to keep current assets productive. When there are exce .ive current assets it is possible that further investments cannot be made, particularly if the current assets are receivables, inventory, or short-term securities. These represent dollars that are tied up in commitments that may be less productive than investment in more services or programs. At Sierra Hospital, the current asset turnover ratio is on the low side, which implies that it has too many current assets. An examination of the balance sheet in Table 3–1 suggests that the assets are excessively linked to accounts receivable. There are also problems of too much cash and excessive miscellaneous current assets. Sierra Hospital needs to convert these assets into a productive capacity.

Fixed Asset Turnover

The fixed asset turnover ratio explores the efficiency of fixed assets in generating revenues:

$$\text{Fixed Asset Turnover (FAT)} = \frac{\text{Total Operating Revenue}}{\text{Total Fixed Assets}}$$

$$\text{Sierra Hospital FAT} = \frac{\$10,097,000}{\$\ 9,098,000} = 1.11$$

A low fixed asset turnover ratio signals that fixed assets are not capable of generating high operating revenues. Since fixed assets refer to investments in plant and equipment *less* accumulated depreciation, there is room for error in interpreting the precise ratios. A high fixed asset ratio will generally imply: (1) the fixed assets are very efficiently managed in generating revenue, or (2) the facilities are very old and highly depreciated, which in turn lowers the revenue needed to compensate for the cost of the assets (i.e., the cost of the assets has been minimized through depreciation). With this perspective it is evident that a new facility will negatively influence the fixed asset turnover ratio because there must be high revenue generation in order to cover the undepreciated cost of the fixed assets.

In the case of Sierra Hospital, its fixed asset turnover ratio is on the low side. The implication is either that the assets are not being used effectively to generate revenue or, more likely in view of the high net income, that the facility and equipment are new and not yet depreciated to any measurable extent. The prognosis is that if Sierra Hospital continues to improve its operating efficiency, it will raise not only net income but the fixed asset ratio as well. Remember that Sierra Hospital also has a plant fund of $516,000. This is a significant reserve that lowers the fixed asset turnover ratio. However, it may not be wise for the hospital to reduce this reserve. Many hospitals currently face problems in replacing fixed assets because they never planned to retain surpluses that would serve as a replacement fund. Now they face very expensive capital due to the high cost of long-term debt and the growing limitations on capital reimbursement by many third party reimbursers.

Inventory Turnover

How long does an inventory of products sit on the shelf of a health care organization before it is completely used up? This question is important because an organization must invest dollars in buying inventory. Yet, as long as the inventory is not used, it is also not earning money. This situation can be tolerated when a certain product today will cost much more money a year from now, more than if the money to purchase the product had been invested in a short-term security. For instance, if the cost of a gross of pharmaceuticals will rise from $560 to $1,080 in one year, and the goods will still be well within their shelf life (i.e., not yet spoiled), then it is better to buy the inventory now than save the $560 in a demand deposit account earning 7.89 percent interest. Such investments in inventory seldom pay off, because price inflation is offset by storage, handling, theft, and spoilage costs.

The issue of inventory turnover is critical when a corporation produces goods. It cannot afford to let inventory become excessive because there is cash invested in the production of goods. The same is true for health care organizations, only to a lesser degree. Excessive inventory implies that management has not introduced an ordering system that minimizes inventory costs.

The calculation of the inventory turnover ratio again uses total operating revenue as a basis for evaluation:

$$\text{Inventory Turnover (IT)} = \frac{\text{Total Operating Revenue}}{\text{Inventory}}$$

$$\text{Sierra Hospital IT} = \frac{\$10,097,000}{\$301,000} = 33.54$$

A high inventory turnover ratio suggests that inventories are turning over rapidly. A low ratio indicates that the organization has invested a large amount of resources in inventory relative to revenue, or that some inventory items may be overstocked. In the case of Sierra Hospital the inventory turnover ratio is somewhat low, but acceptable given the nature of health care organizations. From all appearances, Sierra Hospital could conceivably reduce the amount of its inventory and still provide needed services.

Leverage Ratios

Leverage ratios are used to assess the strength of an organization's capital position. These ratios reflect the extent of debt maintained by the firm. As a result there is a direct relation to the ability to service both short- and long-run obligations. Among the salient features of the leverage ratios are the following:

- The ratios convey the extent to which resources are tied up in long-term debt and short-term debt.
- Excessive long-term debt implies lower liquidity.

- The ratios reflect the ability to pay fixed charges and payments (e.g., principal and interest payments).
- Excessive long-term debt implies an inability to handle unforeseen contingencies such as liquidations or malpractice suits (assuming that the award of a suit is more than the hospital is insured for).
- Leverage ratios will influence bond ratings and hence make tax-exempt revenue bonds for hospital construction more or less marketable depending on existing leverage.

It is apparent in the preceding points that the leverage ratios have much to do with the long-term financing aspects of a health care facility. As such, these ratios capture the essence of financial management as the basis for lending and borrowing funds for construction, renovation, or expansion of facilities.

Debt to Total Assets

The debt ratio or ratio of long-term debt to total assets is a standard used in corporations to assess their borrowing capacity:

$$\text{Debt to Total Assets (DTA)} = \frac{\text{Long-Term Debt}}{\text{Total Assets}}$$

$$\text{Sierra Hospital DTA} = \frac{\$\,4,412,000}{\$13,113,000} = .34$$

As the ratio suggests, when total debt is high relative to total assets, the figure is also high; when an organization has a low amount of debt, then the debt ratio approaches zero. Obviously, if an organization does not have an extensive level of debt it is in a good position to borrow money (to increase its leverage) because it does not have any commitments that it must honor. When the debt ratio is high, then the organization has many obligations to honor.

Total assets enter the picture in terms of the security that an organization can document. With a low debt ratio there are many assets to the level of debt. Thus default is unlikely, and if it did occur, the creditors would be able to retrieve their funds by litigation over the existing assets. The assets serve as security for an uncertain investment. Since virtually all investments include a portion of risk, the debt ratio helps to assess the level of risk. Such risk may not be entirely a problem in health care organizations given the availability of third party revenue and the relatively inelastic demand for medical care. However, high competition and prospective payment all serve to jeopardize the formerly low risk of investments in hospitals.

Sierra Hospital has a debt to total assets ratio of .34, which suggests that the hospital has not overused debt to acquire its existing assets. The hospital has considerable flexibility remaining to borrow long-term debt if it needs to acquire other facilities or plant or cover some other expense area. The implication is that Sierra Hospital is using a minimal amount of financial leverage to cover its operations. From a risk perspective the implication is that Sierra Hospital does not have to worry about covering its current or future obligations. There is sufficient flexibility left to borrow funds using long-term debt.

Times Interest Earned

Since the largest portion of most debt payments includes the interest to be paid on a mortgage or bond, the financial officer is concerned with the times interest earned ratio. This ratio involves the earnings before taxes and captures the ability of a health care organization to service the interest portion of debt out of current earnings. As the ratio increases, the ability of the organization to pay its interest expense also increases. Therefore it is critical that organizations manage their debt and revenue such that the interest portion can be easily serviced.

The times interest earned ratio is calculated as:

$$\text{Times Interest Earned (TIE)} = \frac{\text{Net Income} + \text{Interest}}{\text{Interest}}$$

$$\text{Sierra Hospital TIE} = \frac{\$2,695,000 + 75,000}{\$75,000} = 36.9$$

It should be apparent that Sierra Hospital has performed excellently in terms of the times interest earned ratio. This is due mainly to the low amount of interest it is paying, as well as the high amount of net income it is clearing. Note that Sierra Hospital pays only $75,000 a year in interest on mortgage bonds of $2,733,000 and $1,679,000. This computes as less than two percent simple interest per year on these obligations. This low interest expense may be possible because Sierra Hospital has only recently acquired the long-term liabilities to pay for new facilities or equipment. It appears that outstanding debt will be easily paid in the future because of the high amount of net income. Remember, however, that the income statement and balance sheet for Sierra Hospital represent only one point in time. Therefore it is best to acquire a longitudinal set of data before concluding that Sierra Hospital is without problems for the future.

Debt to Equity

The debt to equity, or debt to fund balance, ratio represents the ratio of long-term debt to the existing equity invested in an organization. The higher the amount of debt the higher will be the ratio. Equity represents the investment made by the owners of all organizations. In nonprofit health care organizations, the concept of equity is replaced by fund balance, but the relationship is still the same. An organization begins to experience difficulty when its debt is more than the equity invested because the debt is not secure. As long as debt is less than equity then lenders are confident that they can acquire their invested funds (e.g., in the form of the loan) from the existing asset base.

The debt to equity ratio is calculated as:

$$\text{Debt to Equity (DTE)} = \frac{\text{Long-Term Debt}}{\text{Equity}}$$

$$\text{Sierra Hospital DTE} = \frac{\$4,412,000}{\$7,564,000} = .58$$

Note that 58 percent of the equity of Sierra Hospital is matched by debt. In another way of viewing this relationship, over 42 percent of all equity in Sierra Hospital is not covered by long-term debt. This percentage of the fund balance can be used to acquire further long-term debt in the sense that there is ample collateral available in the form of owners' equity. The stockholders (or trustees) have an increasing interest to make certain that debt is minimized under these conditions in order that the hospital can continue to perform successfully.

Total Assets to Equity

Another important ratio that conveys the extent of financial leverage is the total assets to equity ratio. This ratio essentially portrays the relationship between assets and equity. When the ratio is high the implication is that the organization is using debt financing to a greater extent. This relationship is readily apparent in its calculations:

$$\text{Total Assets to Equity (TAE)} = \frac{\text{Total Assets}}{\text{Equity}}$$

$$\text{Sierra Hospital TAE} = \frac{\$13,113,000}{\$7,564,000} = 1.73$$

How does debt enter into the equation? The total assets figure must vary with the amount of debt acquired to purchase new assets, or with debt such as accounts payable that are used to produce a good or service. There is a close association between the total assets to equity ratio and debt financing.

The total assets to equity ratio for Sierra Hospital suggests that a very low amount of debt financing is being used relative to the total equity. Therefore Sierra Hospital is in a position of considerable strength to avoid default.

USING RATIOS

As we have seen, the calculation of financial ratios is a convenient beginning for analyzing the financial performance of a health care organization. However, it is important to underscore the fact that the calculation of ratios is only a beginning from which further analysis should proceed. Like any index or construct, the ratios have most value when they are compared with certain standards. In the case of business corporations and health care organizations this means that there must be some aggregated source of data. This can occur in at least two forms: (1) longitudinal analysis of a firm's set of financial ratios and (2) ratios that are calculated for an entire industry.

Before considering both of these means for analyzing ratios, it is appropriate to underscore the fact that financial ratios are best understood in relation to themselves. Hence a series of profitability ratios have greatest meaning when they are compared with the same ratios over the same time period. Ratios also have more meaning when compared with one another. In this sense, the corporation may discover that its profitability ratios are decreasing. At the same time the liquidity ratios may indicate that the problem is basically one of accounts receivable and cash flow during the reporting period. Therefore nurse administrators and other health care managers should be concerned about calculating more than just a ratio. They should also be concerned with how those ratios compare over time in order to provide an accurate portrait of the organization.

Longitudinal Analysis

The longitudinal analysis of a health care organization's financial ratios assumes:

- the methods of accounting for key variables have remained constant,
- the fiscal period has not changed,
- financial data and records have been retained over time,
- the organization has not experienced a crisis such that interpretation of ratios is meaningless,
- management will actually implement strategies needed to improve the financial ratios, and

- significant environmental problems (e.g., inflation) have not affected the data.

Sierra Hospital can serve as an illustration. Assume that it has attained the following levels of performance on the ratios over the last three years:

	Earliest *Year 1*	*Year 2*	*Most Recent* *Year 3*
Return on Equity	.12	.21	.36
Return on Total Assets	.10	.15	.21
Debt to Equity	.83	.62	.58
Average Payment Period	70.6	60.7	50.9
Days in Accounts Receivable	102.7	110.9	102.5

Several years' data are very helpful in seeing trends within each ratio and among the ratios. Overall it appears that Sierra Hospital has gradually been improving its financial performance. The question that remains is why?

The profitability ratios of return on equity and return on total assets show impressive gains over the three years. Hence profitability is a result of something more than just fluctuations in the asset or equity base. The debt to equity ratio implies that the high level of performance in the profitability ratio may be due to rapidly decreasing levels of debt. The capacity to pay off long-term debt must in some manner be related to patient revenues. The liquidity ratio for days in accounts receivable suggests that Sierra Hospital has been able to consistently achieve significant reductions in the length of time required to receive payment on charges.

Exactly why the receivables are being paid earlier is not ascertainable from the data. But, *the ratios serve as a foundation for further inquiry*. Perhaps it is ongoing negotiations with third party payers to process their claims earlier. Perhaps it is a new prepayment policy with a retrospective adjustment policy for payment by a major third party payer. Alternatively, perhaps the hospital has enforced a new collections program. Whatever the reason, the ratios furnish the health care manager with a foundation from which investigation can commence. This investigation should take note of the change in the average payment period. However, in all likelihood this ratio has changed as a result of a reduced time to obtain receivables. By analytically comparing the financial ratios of Sierra Hospital, health care managers are in a better position to assess the financial management policies of the organization.

A longitudinal analysis for the Humana Corporation is shown in Table 3–3. The financial ratios cover the ten-year period from 1974 to 1983. Generally the ratios show good performance on the part of Humana. There are consistent improvements in all ratios: activity, profitability, leverage, and liquidity. It is interesting to

Table 3-3 Ratio Analysis for Humana Corporation

RATIO	1974	1975	1976	1977	1978	1979	1980	1981	1982	1983
Current	1.46	1.36	1.41	1.52	1.53	1.49	1.39	1.41	1.56	1.71
Quick	1.28	1.15	1.23	1.36	1.39	1.35	1.25	1.31	1.43	1.58
ACP	88.13	63.81	62.76	58.29	65.80	44.88	41.40	40.12	39.76	40.88
Inv. Turn	23.79	24.99	33.63	37.98	34.94	33.38	39.27	44.81	44.18	41.34
Ar. Turn	4.09	5.64	5.74	6.17	5.47	8.02	8.70	8.97	9.04	8.81
TA Turn (%)	.50	.63	.77	.81	.68	.78	.84	.89	.87	.80
Fixed Asset Turn	.62	.75	.94	1.03	.85	.98	1.07	1.21	1.15	1.04
Gross Profit	22.60	21.40	21.90	23.20	24.90	21.40	22.60	22.50	23.60	25.60
Net Profit	3.05	1.97	2.10	3.17	4.73	4.41	5.78	6.94	8.39	9.10
ROE	6.90	5.71	7.30	11.94	18.30	17.40	22.90	25.80	25.10	24.00
RO Common	6.93	5.80	7.41	11.94	25.64	19.62	26.35	23.30	31.21	25.33
ROA	1.56	1.23	1.60	2.56	3.19	3.44	4.87	6.20	7.20	7.24
TIE	2.17	1.59	1.76	2.05	2.31	2.01	2.34	2.92	3.28	3.30
Debt Ratio (%)	.78	.79	.79	.78	.83	.75	.79	.76	.74	.70
Debt/Equity	3.45	3.69	3.65	3.58	4.73	3.81	3.70	2.65	2.92	2.31
Debt as % of Total Cap.	.74	.76	.75	.75	.80	.77	.75	.67	.70	.65

Sources: Annual Report, Humana Corporation, 1983; "Humana," Value Line Investment Survey, Value Line Inc., © January 1985.

note that Humana has been able to decrease its debt while raising its profitability. Overall, the ten-year performance analysis suggests that management has been implementing the necessary adjustments to support continued improvement. It is only with the availability of the longitudinal analysis that a more complete understanding of where this firm has been and where it is going can be derived.

Industry Analysis

Industry analysis is predicated on a set of financial ratios that have been calculated for all organizations of a similar type. For example, the American Hospital Association and the Healthcare Financial Management Association periodically collect data that facilitate computation of ratios. In this manner a given health care organization can be compared with others with similar goals. For example, nonprofit hospitals can be contrasted with other nonprofit hospitals. These comparisons have several advantages:

- They provide ratios on many facilities.
- The data are available over several years' performance.
- The ratios provide a standard for comparison.
- It is possible to ascertain trends in specific ratios.
- Objective evidence provided in the ratios removes the subjectivity inherent in assessing a given set of ratios for a single hospital.

The comparisons also have several disadvantages:

- The data are provided by many hospitals; hence there is little control over how accounting measures are used or how financial variables are interpreted.
- There is room for error in the aggregation and calculation of data.
- There is no true basis of comparison for a hospital because each hospital faces a different environment.

A wise reading of these advantages and disadvantages suggests that it is best to use industry ratios as a supplement to the assessment of a given organization's set of ratios. Such comparisons should not represent the final standard by which a hospital or health care organization's ratios are evaluated.

Table 3–4 presents an industry analysis of comparative financial ratios for major health care corporations in 1983. These ratios are meant to illustrate the variability among the industry's leaders. Note that the net profit margin varies from 5.3 to 9.1 percent. Yet this 172 percent difference is lessened when we consider the total capital invested. The main point in Table 3–4 is that there are variations in financial ratios even among corporations of similar size in the same industry.

Table 3–4 Comparative Financial Ratios of Major Health Care Corporations, 1983

COMPANY	Operating Margin	Net Profit Margin	Return on Total Capital	Return on Net Worth	LTD as % of Total Capital (1982)	Return on Total Assets	Current Ratio
American Medical International	22.6	7.6	11.7	21.0	50.6	7.1	1.5
Hospital Corporation of America	20.8	7.6	10.2	15.5	52.8	6.2	1.7
Humana	25.8	9.1	12.7	24.0	62.4	7.9	1.5
National Medical Enterprises	17.5	5.3	9.0	14.3	N/A	5.8	2.3

Sources: *Industry Norms and Key Business Ratios*, Dun and Bradstreet, 1982–1983; "Medical Services Industry," *Value Line Investment Survey*, Value Line Inc., © January 1985; and *Industry Averages*, Standard and Poor, 1984.

Application to Sierra Hospital

To illustrate the use of comparative ratios we can turn again to Sierra Hospital. For our purposes we can consider the 1982 ratios for Hospital Corporation of America (HCA)—one of the large investor-owned hospital chains. The advantage of using HCA is that its data (i.e., financial ratios) are very reliable, since a single corporate information system is involved, and since HCA had more than 370 hospitals in 1982. The ratios for HCA are shown in Table 3–5 along with the ratios for Sierra Hospital.

Some interesting similarities and differences can be summarized as follows:

- Sierra Hospital does not have the liquidity of HCA, although its days in accounts receivable and average payment period ratios are lower.

Table 3–5 Comparative Assessment of Financial Performance

Ratio	Hospital Corporation of America 1982	Sierra Hospital
Liquidity		
Current Ratio	6.62	3.5
Acid Test	4.48	3.3
Days in Accounts Receivable	121.38	102.5
Average Payment Period	98.14	50.9
Days Cash on Hand	439.20	12.2
Profitability		
Return on Equity (Fund Balance)	.12	.36
Return on Total Assets	.10	.21
Operating Margin	.12	.17
Nonoperating Revenue	.48	.35
Discounts and Allowances	N/A	.05
Activity		
Total Asset Turnover	.64	.77
Current Asset Turnover	.68	2.15
Fixed Asset Turnover	11.47	1.11
Inventory Turnover	11.29	33.54
Leverage		
Debt to Total Assets	1.18	.34
Times Interest Earned	0.00	36.9
Debt to Equity	.01	.58
Total Assets to Equity	1.18	1.73

Source: Data for Hospital Corporation of America were obtained from *Healthcare Financial Management,* Vol. 37, p. 56, Healthcare Financial Management Association, © December 1983.

- Sierra Hospital is providing a much better return on investment as shown in the profitability ratios.
- The results for the activity ratios are mixed. Sierra Hospital is turning its assets over more often, including inventory, but it is lagging in the fixed asset turnover ratio.
- Sierra Hospital has considerably more leverage than HCA.

Note that the comparative ratios establish a basis for further analysis. They do not answer all the questions about the financial performance of a given health care facility.

SELF STUDY EXERCISES

In order to improve your skills in calculating and interpreting financial ratios, return to the balance sheet, Table 2–1, and income statement, Table 2–4, for data to compute the following ratios. Answers for the correct ratios with a summary interpretation are in Appendix A.

Calculate these ratios:

1. current ratio
2. acid test ratio
3. days in accounts receivable
4. average payment period
5. return on total assets
6. operating margin
7. total asset turnover
8. current asset turnover
9. debt to total assets
10. debt to equity

NOTES

1. Irwin T. David, "Why Tax-exempt Hospitals Need Profit," *Hospital Financial Management* 39 (September 1982): 46–49, 52, 54.
2. "How to Read a Financial Statement," *Trustee* 37 (December 1984): 17–18.
3. James T. Whitman, "Ratio Analysis—Indispensible Management Aid," *Hospital Financial Management* 33 (September 1979): 74.
4. Steven A. Finkler, "Ratio Analysis: Use with Caution," *Health Care Management Review* 7 (Spring 1982): 65–72.
5. Russell A. Caruana and George Kudder, "Seeing Through the Figures with Ratios," *Hospital Financial Management* 32 (June 1978): 16–26.

6. Walter J. Garbarczyk, "Should Hospital Financial Statements Continue to Apply Fund Accounting Principles?" *Hospitals* 52 (November 1, 1978): 49–50.

7. William O. Cleverley and George S. Massar, "How Hospitals Measure Liquidity," *Healthcare Financial Management* 37 (November 1983): 66–72.

8. Doorwin W. Schlag, "How Hospital Finances Affect the Bottom Line," *Hospital Financial Management* 35 (October 1981): 76–79.

9. Bruce R. Neumann and James D. Suver, "ROI: A Diagnostic Tool for a Health Bottom Line," *Hospital Financial Management* 34 (July 1980): 14–18, 21–22.

10. Michael D. Rosko and Robert W. Broyles, "Unintended Consequences of Prospective Payment: Erosion of Hospital Financial Position and Cost Shifting," *Health Care Management Review* 9 (Summer 1984): 35–43.

11. Gene Sandleback, "Financial Ratio Analysis," *Healthcare Financial Management* 37 (January 1983): 61–62.

Chapter 4

Financial Planning, Budgeting, and Control

Of all of the management functions, few have been neglected in health care organizations more than planning, budgeting, and control. These topics are often discussed with religious enthusiasm, but they are also neglected in actual practice. The reasons behind this mistreatment of planning, budgeting, and control are many. However, one factor stands out more than any other as the causal force. There has been no incentive for health care executives to establish effective planning, budgeting, or control systems. As a result, health care organizations have been managed by intuition, incremental decisions, and lack of knowledge about results attained. There has been little if any orientation to managing for performance; that is, to continually improve operations. The main exceptions to this have occurred in organizations driven relentlessly by a dominant goal (e.g., profit) or those that have continually confronted severe constraints (e.g., low reimbursement rates in the nursing home industry).

Nursing administrators must understand this background to planning, budgeting, and control in order to appreciate why many health care organizations are still struggling to raise their performance. Although there are many causal factors, such rudimentary failures exist because reimbursement policies have failed to establish an *incentive* for good performance. Existing in a reimbursement climate that covered almost all costs (i.e., retrospective payment), health care organizations had little motivation to control the costs of service.

Only within the last decade have there been serious policy efforts to control health care costs. The government, working in concert with private insurance carriers, has made substantial inroads in removing the cost-pass-through option for health providers. Copayment, higher deductibles, benefit limitations, means tests, and other cost control mechanisms are now redirecting the incentive system. The spread of prospective payment, prepayment, and capitation systems are improving the odds for control over health expenditures.

In sum, health care organizations have not been motivated in the past to attain efficient resource use. In effect, they have been subsidized by the third party payers and patients (through higher premiums). As long as this climate persisted, there was virtually no reason to devise and implement sound planning, budgeting, and control systems. Although bits and pieces of such systems have been developed within most health care organizations, concern for systems development has been infrequent. In one hospital a strategic planning program may be solidly in place. In another hospital attention may have been directed more toward the accounting side to achieve control over some aspects of operations. In still another facility the hospital may have created sound planning and control components yet overlooked the importance of budgeting as an effective tool for operational planning and control.

Nursing administrators will experience many of the problems that result from poor planning, budgeting, and control systems. They will not know what precise goals or objectives their work units, departments, or organizations are pursuing in some circumstances. In other cases they will be asked to adhere to budgets, but then they will be neither penalized nor rewarded for doing so. It is likely that for all of their conscientiousness in managing their unit of responsibility, nurse administrators will see other health care managers rewarded despite the fact that performance in these other units was actually lower than in the nursing department. Because of this state of affairs, the links between the pieces may not be obvious. Nurse administrators may have a difficult time trying to understand how all of the smaller pieces—goals, objectives, budgets, planning calendars, monthly performance reviews, audits, and so forth—fit together in an integrated and comprehensible whole. Consequently it will be difficult to lead staff members toward better performance when the managerial system fails to provide needed guidance and support.

However, as long as nurse administrators are cognizant of what constitute ideal models of planning, budgeting, and control, and are adept at constructively identifying the weaknesses of these systems within their organizations, they will make a solid contribution to management. Financial performance ultimately will be the beneficiary where nurse administrators help to create better planning, budgeting, and control. Benefits should also accrue to many other aspects of the organization's performance. Nurse administrators must function as constructive advocates who help health care organizations progress toward better planning, budgeting, and control not only in nursing but in other management areas as well.

THE FINANCING ELEMENTS OF PLANNING, BUDGETING, AND CONTROL

It is important to remember that the finance area is only one aspect of an overall planning, budgeting, and control system. Although the emphasis in this book is on the financial function of nurse administrators, it is important to recognize that this function occurs within a context of human resource management, organization structure, marketing, information processing, operations management, environmental reaction, and numerous other functions. As a result, there is substantial reason to consider the broader context of planning, budgeting, and control.

Synergism among Components

The synergism among planning, budgeting, and control and its relevance for health care organizations has been effectively defined by Vraciu as three essential phases in an integrated management control system.[1] In our view it is the planning phase and its operational equivalent—programming—that actually drive any practical model of management control. Without having preestablished desired end results in the form of verifiable goals and objectives, there is literally nothing to control for. There is no standard that can be used to confirm whether performance was good or bad (i.e., lived up to performance expectations). Consequently there is no understanding of whether resources were judiciously managed or whether the organization failed to employ its resources wisely.

Planning provides meaning to both budgeting and control. Budgeting is the operationalization of plans for a specific work unit, department, program, division, or other meaningful organizational component. A budget can also define the intentions of the organization itself. The key to understanding this difference is to recognize the time frame of plans versus budgets. Budgets are usually yearly articulations of plans. Although plans may also be defined in terms of yearly increments, they provide a broad direction of ends to be achieved rather than a specific determination of how resources will be allocated.

Control is the process that identifies deviations from either broad plans or specific budgets. The purpose of management control, therefore, is to identify and correct deviances in performance. Control activities themselves may be adjusted to the time frame of either the plan or budget since control activities maintain a useful application at any point in time. As a result it is possible to depict the interrelationships among planning, budgeting, and control as shown in Figure 4–1. Many authorities suggest that planning leads to budgeting, which in turn leads to control.[2,3] However, as found in the real world, such cycles rarely occur. More often there is incremental effort involving all functions. Seldom does the cycle occur so neatly that at year end (or whatever planning-budgeting time frame) the control process provides a convenient review from which plans are altered for the forthcoming period. This is particularly true at the nursing department level.

Assuming that a plan has been established for the nursing department as part of the strategic planning effort, and that the plan is then articulated in terms of a specific budget, the cycle has begun. A likely scenario is that within a few months' time the controller will be reviewing progress on expenses and revenues. The finance or operations committee may be forced to devise methods for cutting back

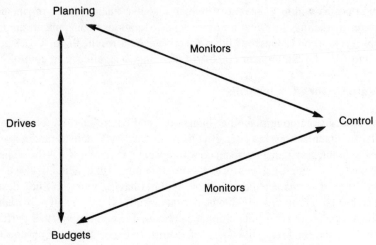

Figure 4–1 The Interrelationships among Planning, Budgeting, and Control

on expenses and for increasing revenues. Many factors may precipitate this effort—declining admissions, restrictions on reimbursement, increases in the cost of supplies, negotiated wages due to a threatened union strike, abnormal turnover among personnel. The health care organization needs action—*control*—now; not later. The well-planned cycle is terminated as the organization shifts to an ad hoc approach. Nursing administrators will recognize this state of affairs. It is more the rule than the exception.

This depiction of the planning, budgeting, and control model is not intended to imply that nursing administrators or other managers should not pursue the ideal model. Quite the contrary; without the pursuit of the ideal it may be difficult if not impossible ever to raise performance. Instead we suggest that nursing administrators look at planning, budgeting, and control from a realistic perspective. The perfect cycle is seldom completed, but it is an end toward which the organization should strive.

Finally, the synergism of the planning, budgeting, and control model should be related to financial management. The setting and attainment of financial goals depends on following through with all components. Setting goals and implementing them in specific budgets are only meaningful when control ensures that dysfunctional deviances do not occur repeatedly or in excessive magnitude.

PLANNING COMPONENT

The hierarchy of plans has been well defined by Steiner, who describes basically three different planning levels:[4]

Planning Level	Time Orientation	Purpose
Strategic	2 years	Determine major goals and objectives for the organization
Medium-Range	1–2 years	Determine specific departmental, divisional, and program plans in order to allocate resources
Short-Range	1 year	Determine budgets to allocate resources during the year

Nursing administrators could be involved at any of these levels depending on their position within the organization and the nature of the organization itself. For example, in a freestanding community hospital that has not diversified its services, a nursing director would participate mainly in medium-range and short-range planning for the nursing department. In other cases the nursing administrator would be asked to participate in institution-wide strategic planning.

When the nursing administrator occupies a corporate staff position that oversees nursing departments in a chain of six hospitals, the opportunities for involvement in strategic planning are more numerous. The nurse administrator may have extensive responsibilities for contributing to all levels of planning within the corporate structure. In contrast, the nursing manager in a small medical group clinic may be involved only in short-range planning. Assuming a staff of five physicians, three registered nurses, and four licensed practical nurses, the head nurse may not be assigned planning responsibilities other than to determine staffing patterns, compensation, and methods for managing nursing turnover (if any) during the coming year.

From a financial management perspective, the levels of planning described above also serve to define a framework for financial planning. Strategic planning for the finance area would involve the determination of major goals and objectives for the organization in the future:

- Establish a rate of return on investment.
- Determine capital investments in plant and major equipment.
- Define markets served and the percentage of each market actually served.
- Establish pricing policies.
- Identify sources of funds (e.g., philanthropy) and a posture for acquiring additional funds.
- Forecast costs, reimbursement changes, capital market trends, and changes in competitors' positions.
- Define accounting and control policies in order to protect assets, identify deviations and discrepancies, and ensure fair financial practices.

Medium-range planning would apply the strategic plans in a more specific and concise fashion at the departmental, divisional, and program level.

Medium-range programming adds specificity to control policies. Instead of broad policies that define the strategic accounting and control plans, medium-range programming elucidates specific performance parameters. An example would be:

Establish Current Operations Policies

- Contribution to return on investment
- Threshold for working capital
- Receivables to current assets
- Current assets to current liabilities
- Operating expenses to total revenue
- Expenses per units of service (e.g., admissions, patient days)

Establish Personnel-Oriented Policies

- Average salary/wage per full-time equivalent
- Payroll as a percent of total revenue
- Revenue per person-hour
- Expenses per person-hour

Establish Patient-Oriented Policies

- Level of bad debt
- Level of charitable care
- Cost per visit/procedure/patient day
- Revenue per visit/procedure/patient day
- Number of patients/procedures served per day

The preceding medium-range plans are meant to be illustrative only. They are not comprehensive in operationalizing the strategic plans nor are they intended to be. There is a hierarchy of plans that becomes increasingly specific as the time frame of planning becomes shorter.

The most obvious time horizon is the short-range planning level. Here the focus is less than one year. Financial plans for this time period include budgets that allocate resources during the year. This is the most important planning activity for most organizational units because the budget translates day-to-day activities into an overall organizational frame of reference. It is the point at which the conceptual is articulated into the specific. Consequently it is also a process that requires very careful attention to make certain that planning guidelines are followed.

A common failure by health care executives at the upper and middle management levels is to overlook the planning aspects of the budget. They may view the budget as only a set of standards that constrain their operations. As a planning document, a budget certainly accomplishes this. However in order to achieve the greatest usefulness, it is essential that budgets are used to help subordinates participate in the planning process. Budgets can establish an overall frame of reference that conveys to employees where their work unit, department, or program is headed. For example, the budget allows nurses to visualize why staffing levels are linked to patient demand for health services. The budget documents that staffing is increased or decreased according to demand. The budget also conveys that a finite set of supplies is available for services. In this manner nurses can cooperate with cost containment plans not only in use of supplies but in other cost-related efforts.

The budget is rarely perceived as a financial plan. Financial management implies more mysterious concepts such as capital budgeting, assessing financial performance, acquiring short-run and long-run capital, or assessing investment opportunities. It is critical that the mysticism surrounding financial management be removed at the earliest possible moment. Budgeting is the basis upon which other financial plans are established and accomplished. In view of this, it is especially important that nursing administrators come to understand the synergism among long-range, medium-range, and short-range plans. Specific budgets should lead inevitably toward long-run financial plans.

Factors Influencing Financial Plans

Nursing administrators should be thoroughly familiar with the factors that influence the creation of financial plans. Among other factors, the more critical determinants of financial plans include market activity, organizational goals, prior performance, trends in third party reimbursement, regulation, competitors' activities, and provider attributes. All of these factors must be incorporated in financial planning. Depending on the planning issue, the nurse administrator should undertake a comprehensive examination that ascertains how each of these factors might influence the creation of a plan or its attainment. In this manner, planning attains a high degree of viability and moves from the conceptual to the applied. It is precisely this step that many executives overlook, and thereby they fail to develop the planning function to meaningfully guide operations.

Market Activity

Market demand for services is an obvious starting point for developing any plan. How many patients are demanding care? In what types of clinical areas is demand highest or lowest? How have these patterns of demand been changing? Is there any association between the level of patient demand and the programmatic efforts by the health care organization? These are only a few of the representative questions that must be answered in formulating a financial plan. The level of patient demand and its direction may be the most essential factor affecting planning because without adequate demand for patient services, there is clearly little reason to anticipate financial gain.

Estimates and direct measures of patient demand have substantial impact at all levels of financial planning. Strategic plans for investment of capital in new facilities or equipment hinge on forecasts of patient demand just as the determination of a yearly budget is related to forecasted demand in a specific service area. Nursing administrators should use the market activity factor as a basis for planning. Either patient demand is sufficient to justify resource allocation or it is not. Planning must be undertaken with this idea firmly in mind.

Organizational Goals

Organizational goals also constrain the number and intended ambitiousness of financial plans. Financial plans are an element of total organizational plans, albeit one of the most essential ingredients. The specific mission, goals, and objectives of the organization should establish a framework for decision making that elucidates directions and prevents unintended investment of resources. These ideas are easy to comprehend, yet many executives fail to use mission statements, goals, or objectives consistently to temper their decision making. As a result the overall outcome is a disjointedness within plans and activities. For example, when the food services department strives to contain costs by purchasing lower grade foodstuffs it may attain the organizational goal of cost control. Simultaneously it may jeopardize other organizational goals that relate to patient amenities or quality of care.

In establishing financial plans there must be direct attention given to organizational goals. Whether the planning process solicits input from trustees, administrative staff, department heads, or managers, it is especially true that financial plans can be correctly tailored to the needs of the organization only if goals are clearly specified. Therefore all organizational members providing input into the planning process should realize that their responsibility is not one to be taken lightly.

Prior Performance

Prior performance establishes a baseline from which future performance targets should be set. The health care organization should remain flexible within that plan to allow deviations in performance; however, there is always a strong need to monitor prior performance. Prior performance should be perceived as a barometer where organizational health is either improving or deteriorating depending on the level of performance attained. There is no better measure of accomplishment than these standards.

Financial planning relies on performance trends to achieve its greatest meaning. Performance is important in all periods of activity, but caution must be used to prevent short-run performance—attainment of gross revenue goals and net income—from dominating the planning process.[5] This tendency to focus on narrow, short-run activities can lead the organization down a fatal path that results in tenuous decisions. The gratification of immediate organizational goals threatens long-run survival.

Trends in Third Party Reimbursement

Trends in third party reimbursement are of interest to every health care executive. The trend is away from cost-pass-through reimbursement toward prospective payment. This means that health care organizations can no longer rely on being paid for just any cost associated with the provision of services. Prospective payment means that health care organizations must plan their activities to guarantee that costs do not exceed payment; otherwise financial solvency will be threatened. This problem is growing as third parties examine prospective payment schemes that pressure health care organizations into cost containment. As reimbursement rates are increasingly constrained by third parties and as payments approach a capitated format, it is clear that health care organizations must respond in both ingenious and conscientious ways.

Health care organizations have tended to respond to prospective payment in two major ways. One strategy is essentially related to financial control while the other addresses expanding the revenue base. Financial control that is designed to contain the costs of providing services has been the dominant strategy of virtually all health care organizations. They seek limits on expenditures by all departments in order to drive down the total cost of care. In the case of Medicare's diagnosis related group payment system, hospitals discovered that they could cut costs in many areas and thereby survive under the financial reimbursement limits. The long-run ramifications of this reaction through cost cutting remain to be seen. However, for the nursing administrator the lesson is very well defined. Financial control of operations has led to more cost-effective performance.

Hospitals have also responded to changes in third party payment by diversifying their services. Hospitals are entering into health care services that traditionally were not linked with acute care institutions. The result is a proliferation of opportunities and a redefinition of what constitutes the hospital. This diversification allows hospitals to tap revenue streams that heretofore were not incorporated within the mainstream of acute care activity. The financial implications are clear. With a high revenue earning capacity, the hospital must plan its diversification very carefully to ensure that an appropriate mix of services is attained. There is a need for planning capital expenditures on plant and equipment and acquisition that transcends normal institutional planning. In sum, changes in third party payment have made the financial planning function more complex.

Regulation

Regulation is a significant factor influencing financial planning in health care organization. Regulation by governmental agencies and professional associations shows no sign of abating in the future and consequently must be factored into long-run financial planning. The main problem is that the health care industry is shifting from a basically laissez-faire economy dominated by a cottage industry of solo practitioners and voluntary nonprofit hospitals to a corporate economy. Unlike other competitive industries, the remarkable fact about the health care system is the extent of third party reimbursement—particularly government involvement through Medicare and Medicaid. After almost twenty years of funding public assistance, national expenditures are more than are budgetarily feasible. This has driven the government and other public and private insurers to seek control of expenditures.

Regulation has gradually gained acceptability as policy within the health system. Beginning with comprehensive health planning, the government has sought to systematically control its expenditures. The certificate of need laws that grew out of health planning were startling to hospitals, nursing homes, and other health care organizations planning major capital investment in either plant or equipment. For the first time, approval had to be acquired from an external regulatory agency prior to purchase of major capital items or initiation of new construction.

These trends in regulation were reinforced and expanded greatly in scope by limits on reimbursement. Allowable reimbursement to hospitals, and fee schedules for physicians, signaled an increasing intensity of regulation that continues today. Prospective payment is an outgrowth of these earlier efforts at control. Regulation of reimbursement through prospective payment has inexorably affected the revenue side of operations. Third party payers are able to control the rate of payment and hence the amount of revenue received by any single health facility. The individual health care organization can only adjust volume and efficiency of inputs. Many health care institutions sought to implement cost control strategies in their management practice, but the revenue side could not be neglected.

Today higher regulatory control implies a need to adjust both revenues and costs in delivery of care. Hence, nursing administrators should understand that financial plans for any multi-institutional system, chain of facilities, facility, department, program, or work unit should address two key strategic elements—revenue enhancement and cost control. It is essential to develop tactics that lower costs (e.g., employee incentive plans for productivity, controls on inventory in supplies and medications, improved staffing patterns, and related operational control measures) while enhancing revenues (e.g., orienting services to specific patient markets such as geriatrics, adolescents, or other meaningful patient-specific market segments, and expanding the scope of services).

Competitors' Activities

Competitors' activities represent another critical variable influencing the financial plans of a health care organization. Almost until the end of the 1970s, overt competition was not respected in the health field. Yet there has always been a subtle form of competition among hospitals based on perceived quality of care. Hospitals tended to congregate in urban locations within close proximity to each other. The distinguishing market features were capacities in specific medical treatment. Under a favorable reimbursement environment this attitude toward competition meshed well with the control of medicine by physicians. The imperative was to provide the highest level of medical care because reimbursement presented few, if any, constraints.

This subtle competition has been replaced by outright aggressiveness among health care organizations. Moreover, competition is being pursued by both for-profit and nonprofit health care organizations. Nonprofit health care organizations have rapidly recognized that they do not have a monopoly on specific services and programs. Without retaliatory competitive responses, they stand a chance of losing not only their advantages in medical specialties, identity in terms of unique equipment, and community respect for philanthropic efforts, but their main revenue base as well.

This dramatic reshaping of the health care market has brought changes in the management of nursing services. Competition will continue to influence the structure and process of nursing services as evidenced by trends for diversification and specialized packaging of nursing care. Competition will also affect recruitment and retention strategies. This in turn influences the nature and extent of financial planning for nursing and other health care services.

Competition forces a greater emphasis on accurately predicting changes in volume. Budgets are contingent on forecasted demand, which can be jeopardized by shifts in patient demand. Not only must health programs undertake greater effort to identify patient demand, they must also develop contingency plans for when demand exceeds or falls short of forecasted levels. This operational financial planning must be adjusted to account for changes in strategy by the health care organization or program. Competition implies modification in current services and budgets; it also implies a strategic response (i.e., new services and promotion that can influence demand) that can increase the need for accuracy in forecasts for patient demand. This effect can become apparent when nurse staffing fails to meet levels of demand, and budgets have been exhausted, leaving little possibility of filling new staff positions or of obtaining slack resources (i.e., through nursing pools).

Provider Attitudes

Provider attitudes represent another key variable influencing financial plans for health care organizations. By provider attitudes we mean the degree to which physicians, nurses, auxiliary personnel, administrators, and other professionals delivering health care services are committed to the organization's financial goals. Commitment to the organization and its goals has been one of the problems confronting nursing administrators and other health care executives.

The current environment of prospective pricing alters the demand for services and hence the demand for professional services. As many hospitals have come to understand, cost control is easily accomplished by cutting the largest cost center— staff salaries and wages. When salaries are reduced there is a corresponding reduction in staffing levels. As a result, some professions such as nursing have contributed more than their share to resolving cost control in hospitals.

Health care organizations continue to view staff as an expendable resource in times of severe budgeting restrictions. The implications for morale and quality patient care are alarming. However, health care facilities are also confronted by the reality that budgets must be met if they are to survive. The financial planning implications are apparent if these trends continue. On one hand nurse administrators will continue to face severe budgetary restrictions on staffing and compensation for good employee performance. On the other hand they will also need to derive the highest possible level of productivity from the existing staff. Commitment to this organizational goal and related financial goals (e.g., cost control and inventory control) may be very difficult to attain.

Nurses will recognize that they are being asked to shoulder the burden of revenue decreases. Staffing levels will decrease, which means more work on their part with less assistance. Fewer resources will be available for raises, basic compensation, and benefits. The health care organization will have less to offer nurses, yet it must ask their commitment to programs that facilitate financial survival. This sort of management environment is exceptionally challenging. Nurse administrators can begin to establish effective management tactics if they realize that the changes are basically financial in origin, and if they consequently help their subordinates comprehend the constraints under which they must operate.

BUDGETING COMPONENT

In financial planning, the strategic planning component is devoted to (1) identifying the primary aims and mission of an organization, program, or department,

(2) establishing a hierarchy of goals and objectives that specify the results to be accomplished, (3) assessing current resources for their ability to help the organization accomplish the targeted end results, and (4) identifying specific programs (e.g., clinical specialties and subspecialties, support programs, or other division of activities) that will be allocated the resources to accomplish the end results. Strategically, the last two elements of the planning process are vital to health care organizations, because in a rapidly changing context it is especially important to determine that expenditures are targeted toward the most viable opportunities.

Tactical or operational planning begins with clearly established strategic plans. Budgeting forms the tactical or operational element of the planning process.[6] In this sense, it addresses the detailed allocation of resources. It is different from strategic planning because budgeting focuses on daily operations and specific resource allocations within a one-year period. By contrast, strategic planning focuses on resource commitments greater than one year. From a financial planning viewpoint, budgeting is directed toward specific resource allocations. It establishes a working articulation of overall strategic plans.

In sum, it is possible to depict financial planning as:

$$\text{financial planning} = \text{strategic plans} + \text{tactical plans}$$

where tactical plans are defined through budgets. This equation depends on full completion of both strategic and tactical elements in order to derive a satisfactory financial plan. Health care and nursing administrators can go awry by overlooking the interrelationship of strategic and tactical plans. Both are essential to good financial planning. Poor planning for facilities (e.g., construction of needed beds) will eventually affect current operations, while poor attention to meeting the budgeted targets for expenditures will threaten the systematic management of the health care institution.

Budgeting Ingredients

There are many different budgets and uses for budgets that nursing administrators need to be cognizant of in the management of their organizations. Nursing administrators should especially be attuned to the different types of budgets because they will interface with most budgeting components of an organization's planning process. Hence, nurse administrators are responsible for working with the financial staff in translating budget objectives into realistic targets in the nursing area.[7]

The first step in developing proficiency in budgeting is to understand the different types of budgets that constitute this component of financial planning. Fundamental to this understanding is an awareness of what budgets actually consist of:

- Specific definitions of plans for operations that are conveyed in essentially quantitative or monetary terms in accordance with projections of demand
- A planned course of action for the year for achieving prespecified goals and objectives, which when accomplished have helped implement a portion of a strategic plan
- Standards and criteria for assessing the effectiveness of expenditures that have been made to meet utilization forecasts

It is valuable for nursing administrators to realize that budgets are no less important than strategic plans even though they have more extensive detail. Although budgets may lack the glamour of the strategic planning level, they are more essential to the financial well-being of a program or organization. Without successful budgeting, the prognosis for achievement of long-run plans is dubious.

Given the definition of budgets elucidated above, ingredients of the budgeting component are shown in Table 4–1. As this outline indicates, master budgets are composed of at least three main ingredients—capital budgets, operating budgets, and cash budgets. All are vital to the financial planning function even though they have varied applicability at the strategic and tactical levels. The capital budget involves long-run financial planning for acquisition, retention, maintenance, and disbursement of major assets for either plant or equipment. As such, this involves a strategic planning orientation. However, it is vital to realize that the tactical budgets—the operating budget and cash budget—are just as important in financial planning even though they occur at the tactical level and are highly concerned with detail.

Estimating Demand

At the tactical level of financial planning demand must be correctly estimated in order to ascertain the health care organization's capacity to fill that demand. If capacity is greater than the demand, this will imply that slack resources exist. For example, a urology ward in a hospital may not be able to maintain more than 65 percent occupancy. Consequently the beds are not being used to capacity. Since these beds are relatively fixed assets, there may be few options available for converting them to better use. However, in terms of the operating budget it is vital not to exceed the required level of staffing.

Although estimates of demand are best defined in terms of a specific competitive setting, the goals of a service-oriented program, and the resources available to serve that demand, it is possible to establish a few general guidelines for estimating demand:[8]

- Segment the population to identify the most likely consumers of the product or service.

Table 4–1 Components of Annual Master Budget

Budgeting Level	Type of Budget	Purpose of Budget
Strategic	Capital Budget	1. Establish a periodic schedule for the disbursement of funds for capital expenditures 2. Determine an operationally acceptable time for the disposal of assets during the year 3. Establish a mechanism for acquiring new resources and for integrating these resources into a schedule for amortization
Tactical	Operating Budget	1. Project estimates of program and facility use through analysis of utilization statistics 2. Project estimates of expenditures in all organizational units 3. Project estimates of anticipated revenue from all sources
Tactical	Cash Flow Budget	1. Estimate the timing of all cash receipts 2. Establish a schedule for all cash disbursements 3. Develop plans for acquiring additional funds during periods of heavy disbursement and for temporarily investing funds during periods of cash reserves

- Estimate the extent to which the program will be able to penetrate the target market segments both before and after promotional efforts or introduction of new services that might directly influence demand.
- Compute the rates at which individuals in the target market segments will encounter (or actually demand) services.
- Develop a monthly forecast for the fiscal year that translates these encounters into service units (e.g., into diagnosis related groups, packages of services, subspecialties, or other convenient category types that are commensurate with the program).
- Estimate the number of encounters that will result due to unexplained variance (i.e., demand that results without an ability to predict its occurrence or cannot be attributed to programmatic efforts).
- Summarize total encounters.

Nurse administrators must familiarize themselves with the methods used by their organizations to forecast demand and utilization.[9] All other tactical and strategic plans build from the estimates of demand. The estimates, therefore, are often the weakest link in financial planning.

CONTROL COMPONENT

Effective operations control should center around at least four components: (1) participation, (2) accountability, (3) performance appraisal, and (4) correction of deficiencies. Although these four concepts seem simple, they are often neglected in many health care organizations.

In recent years there has been greater pressure to devise and implement functional control systems that are oriented toward finances and performance. Although some nursing administrators may not be directly responsible for creating an overall control program, they do have responsibility for working with other health care managers in designing a control system. A valuable element of this design is a financial orientation to decision making. Since nurse administrators are directly involved in the tactical aspects of financial planning—particularly budgeting—it is only appropriate that they help to emphasize the need to create effective control mechanisms. These mechanisms consist of four key ideas.

Participation

The best control is direct control; that is, control implemented by the person who is performing a job or service. This implies that all nursing staff must participate in controlling performance, whether holding down costs or delivering quality care. From a financial management perspective, nurses must be integrated into the cost control program of a health facility. They must actively participate in keeping costs to a minimum. Without this collaborative effort the end result will be higher costs. Nursing administrators recognize that it is the staff nurse who is ultimately responsible for controlling costs. Supervisors cannot, and should not, attempt to control every action of their staff members. There is only one viable alternative, and this is to elicit participation on the part of all nursing staff members.

There are many mechanisms for attaining participation:

- developing a team atmosphere through collaborative practice
- offering incentives that are attached to a system of specifically attained goals (e.g., salary increases dependent on budget targets achieved)

- selecting nurses (after employment interviews) who have the same goals as the health facility (e.g., who are interested in an association with the organization beyond individual goals of salary or mere employment)
- integrating financially oriented goal accomplishment with professional identity

The important part of these and other mechanisms for eliciting participation is that nurses are recognized as the prime movers in controlling performance. Their unit managers or leaders may have responsibility for overall control, but it is the staff nurse who ultimately determines whether broad financial goals of the organization are attained.

Accountability

Control is established where individuals are held accountable for accomplishing various goals. This has been a critical problem in health care control. Organizations have generally failed to hold staff accountable for their performance; as a result mediocre performance was tolerated in many areas. Although there has always been a compelling commitment to excellence in the delivery of medical care, there has also been a corresponding failure to make a commitment to financially oriented performance. Health care organizations are now challenged to expand the expectations of staff in terms of financial performance.

Accountability may include:

- refusing to award raises for less than exemplary performance
- terminating staff who consistently fail to contribute to financial goals such as cost control
- promoting staff who have demonstrated a capacity to lead others in the attainment of basic financial goals
- identifying and rewarding staff who perform at an outstanding level

These are only a few of the methods that nurse administrators can use in developing their programs of control. The key to controlling financial performance is to hold personnel accountable.

Performance Appraisal

If a nurse administrator expects to hold personnel accountable for attaining financially related goals, then it is imperative to appraise performance. How can staff be held accountable unless the effort expended and the goals accomplished have been assessed? Unfortunately there are few effective performance appraisal systems functioning in the health care field. The reason for this deficiency relates again to the nature of retrospective reimbursement. Fortunately health care organizations are now cognizant of the need to create effectively functioning appraisal systems that accurately measure performance.

Within the assessment criteria, attention should be directed toward financial goals in the nursing program, department, or work unit. The evaluation criteria must specify the financial performance desired (e.g., inventory control, budgeting milestones achieved, or services delivered per diem). Nurses should be alerted to these criteria and should participate in their formation and specification. If desired end results are not specified, it will be very difficult to measure the accomplishment of these objectives.

Correction of Deficiencies

The final control component is the correction of deficiencies. Once participation has been attained, accountability implemented and performance evaluated, it is essential that any deficiencies be corrected. The ability to correct deficiencies depends on the extent to which an organization supports and tolerates change. For example, assume that a nurse administrator wants her organization to implement a variable billing system centered on patient classification.[10] The purpose of the billing system is to determine a more accurate charge per patient for nursing services. Unless the organization supports change (i.e., introduction of the new billing system), it is unlikely that patient charges will reflect true nursing costs.

In terms of financial management, the correction of deficiencies is often easier said than done. A complex number of factors ultimately drive the financial performance of any program or organization. From the nurse administrator's perspective it is vital that this fact be recognized. It is very difficult to ascertain cause and effect, much less to implement a program designed to manipulate relevant variables. Nurse administrators can expect to function as advocates for change— this may mean working with others in identifying the causes of budget overruns and in seeking solutions. This openness to collaborating with others can contribute positively toward financial performance.

FINANCIAL FORECASTING

Many health care managers believe that they cannot afford the luxury of planning because they are too busy addressing one crisis after another. Although forecasting demand and utilization is the cornerstone of financial planning, health care executives spend even less time forecasting for future demand than in planning for current projects and operations. What they may fail to recognize is that an unplanned project often takes many times longer to complete than expected, or that the failure to anticipate higher demand causes substantial difficulties. A carefully planned program that has accurately forecasted demand can avoid many of these problems.[11] By adjusting the operations schedule to satisfy what would have been unforecasted demands, services will be produced, goals will be achieved, and maximum profits or minimum costs are more likely to result.

Nursing administrators must continue to forecast even though they realize that their forecast probably will be inaccurate due to factors beyond their control.[12] In financial planning it is the *process* of forecasting that is beneficial. Forecasting usually involves subjective or objective approaches to predicting future values. The subjective approach incorporates the opinions or judgments of one or more persons who are experienced or considered knowledgeable. Objective procedures focus on using quantitative techniques to project past values into the future. Both of these approaches should be integrated into the forecasting process.

The first step in financial forecasting is to establish the purpose for developing the forecast; there are many valid managerial uses of a forecast. Forecasts of next year's services in the obstetrics unit could be used by the nursing administrator to establish scheduling patterns for nurse midwives or to make budgeting decisions for the supplies used by the unit in alternative birthing packages of care. An optimistic demand forecast might be inappropriate for the realistic cost-minimizing implementation of collaborative practice. Hence, many health care organizations develop separate forecasts for different purposes in the financial planning function—demand projections, expenses in operations management, and revenue sources.

Financial forecasting also involves collecting and displaying relevant historical data to determine if any patterns would help in predicting future values. Since the intent is to identify trends, seasons, or cycles associated with the past that could be projected into the future, historical data should be cleansed of any one-time occurrences that probably will not reoccur in the future. Data are commonly obtained from organizational records. Since graphical displays often reveal underlying regularities in past demand or performance levels, plotting the past data over time may provide a visual understanding that surpasses analysis by other more sophisticated quantitative methods. Particularly in the financial management area, there are often tendencies to overanalyze data through sophisticated quantitative techniques. Nurse administrators need to be judicious in their use of these techniques especially when there is the need to communicate these ideas and results to others.

Consideration should be given to using one or more of the three main types of forecasting models in financial planning. The models have their unique characteristics, but they all can be used for a variety of managerial situations. Time series models use an item's own historical data to predict future demand. For example, the historical demand for Demerol can be used to forecast the demand for pharmaceuticals during inpatient care. Specific techniques within each time series model may be as simple as an arithmetic average or as complex as multiple regression. These quantitative techniques are all based on the assumption that the future will continue to be like the past.[13]

Subjective models are more qualitative in nature, bringing together expert opinion and any other information that may relate to the usually nonextractable, distinct future behavior of the item being forecasted. For example, a panel of nurse administrators may be used to forecast the trends in salaries for licensed practical nurses—the managerial expertise is used as an informed opinion in developing a budget for staff nurses.

The summary of forecasting methods found in Table 4–2 illustrates the analytical foundations for a financial plan.

The specific technique(s) that minimize forecast error should be selected. Additional tests should be run to see how accurately various techniques have predicted actual values during the past 6–12 months. A practical approach is to select that technique that has the smallest average forecast error and use it to forecast over the next planning horizon—short term (1–3 months) or intermediate term (3–24 months). Long-term forecasts often require agreements between members of an expert panel in selecting a satisfactory approach. The chosen technique should be sufficiently accurate, of reasonable cost, and most importantly, easily understood by those using it.

The nurse administrator must also incorporate the impact of appropriate internal and external factors on the output of the forecast model. Estimates of influence of new program services, marketing promotions, price changes, or service upgrades need to be converted into quantitative adjustments. Changes in the demand cycle, new government regulations, or anticipated activities of competitors and other environmental activities must be evaluated to assess their impact on the forecasted value. Managerial judgment is required to determine the impact of these factors on the projected forecast.

Table 4–2 Forecasting Methods Relevant to Financial Planning

Characteristic	Time Series Model	Causal Model	Subjective Model
Relative Cost	Very Low	Moderate	High
Technology Needed	Calculator	Computer with statistical software	None
Forecast Horizon	Short Term (1–3 Months)	Intermediate Term (3–24 Months)	Long Term (2–10 Years)
Typical Applications	Inventory Control	Demand Projections	Reimbursement Policies

It is vital to document all assumptions and rationales underlying the forecasting process. While a written report serves as a record of what was done and why, the real benefit occurs when the process is successful and documentation is readily available to replicate the forecasting procedures for the next planning period.

Finally, every nurse administrator needs to continually monitor the forecast error and decide whether the process is producing an acceptable forecast for planning purposes. If the error rate is tolerable, then the forecast should be updated for the next planning period. If not, a new forecast model or a specific technique may be needed.

In short, the benefits of better understanding and greater sensitivity to the operations and environment of a health care organization accrue to those who engage in the forecasting process. This activity is especially needed in financial planning. The basis for most financial plans—capital budgets, cash budgets, and operating budgets—are constructed upon estimates of demand. Financial forecasting must create accurate and reliable demand or utilization estimates. Once this parameter is established, it is possible to formulate specific tactical and strategic elements of a health care organization's financial plans. Nurse administrators should be actively involved in this process and should possess a fundamental knowledge of the purpose and interrelationships in forecasting and planning even though they may not be thoroughly versed in the specific forecasting techniques themselves.

INFORMATION SYSTEMS SUPPORTING FINANCIAL PLANNING

Most nursing administrators recognize that they need good information to enhance their effectiveness in making decisions and in financial planning. Information is used at all financial planning steps within a health care organization and by all departments. Development of a meaningful plan to improve departmental, program, or organizational performance requires quality information. Superior financial planning to secure that performance is supported by the availability of relevant, useful, and accurate information. Without appropriate information, the performance of every health care executive is impaired.

Current Trends in Information Systems

Recently, changes in the competitive environment of health care organizations have led to an increase in the demand for information.[14] Financial planning by nurse administrators and other health care managers requires accessible and timely information to develop effective, cost-efficient plans for action in the face of such a changing environment.

In the past, health care organizations have developed management systems, both manual and computer-based, to assist them in meeting demands for information. Many systems have been implemented to provide operational level control functions, including patient billing and collections, payroll, inventory, purchasing and receiving, patient registration, personnel, and service scheduling.[15,16] Management systems have been developed to support information storage, retrieval, and processing for routine, repetitive decision making and planning purposes. Still other systems have been built to provide flexible, user-directed modeling capabilities for nonroutine, ad hoc decision making and planning. Applications include budget preparation and analysis, capital expenditure decisions, cost containment and productivity analysis, diagnosis related group reimbursement modeling, and clinical diagnosis.[17]

More emphasis is now being placed on developing information systems that mimic the performance of an ''expert'' in a particular field of endeavor. Notable successes have been achieved in medical diagnosis and consultation systems for assisting physicians in clinical management.[18-23] While they have been slow to permeate managerial application areas, such systems are just as applicable to financial planning functions and other strategic management activities that require expertise and informed judgment.

The importance of computer-based management systems to nursing services and health care organizations varies with each organization.[24] For some, information system activities represent an area of great strategic importance, while for others they will always play a cost-effective and useful but distinctly supporting role.[25] In many cases, the strategic application of information system technology can even provide a health care organization with a distinct competitive advantage. Computer-based management systems can help formulate and execute appropriate competitive strategies, such as becoming the low-cost provider for a given service, differentiating its care offerings from competing hospitals or health care facilities, or identifying and filling the needs of a specially defined patient market niche.[26-28]

Overview of Computerized Information Systems

Recent and continuing advances in information processing technology, coupled with the growth in application complexity, have stimulated a corresponding evolution in computer-based management systems. Four basic types of systems have evolved during the past three decades: electronic data processing (EDP) systems, management information systems (MIS), decision support systems (DSS), and expert systems (ES). All of these systems can apply to the financial planning function, yet some are more appropriate than others.

Electronic data processing (EDP) systems were introduced to perform data storage, retrieval, and transaction processing. As the emphasis shifted from clerical processing toward providing information to managers in functional areas of the organization, the systems came to be known as management information systems (MIS). Systems that document nursing costs usually fall in the category of MIS.[29] Later, emphasis on a decision-centered approach to the development of information systems led to a class of systems referred to as decision support systems (DSS). More recently, problem-solving programs designed to perform difficult, domain-specific tasks at a high level of performance have brought expert systems (ES) to the forefront.

In terms of applicability to financial planning in most health care organizations and systems, the EDP and MIS systems are the most widely available. Nurse administrators may discover some DSS applications, but at the moment most health care organizations have so concentrated on processing data (e.g., patient records and patient bills) that they have not progressed toward relating the data to decisions.

Electronic Data Processing (EDP)

These computer-based systems help achieve operational control by automating structured clerical tasks. The EDP system typically automates routine transaction processing, record storage and retrieval, and report generation as part of a larger management system. These systems have wide application in health care financial functions. General ledger transaction processing, inventory order determination, and clinic appointments are representative of applied EDP systems. In spite of the highly structured nature of many of these applications, the EDP system rarely facilitates control of the organizational system with which it interacts.

The principal components of an EDP system usually include data collection procedures and a library of programs for data manipulation. These features make EDP perfect for managing the basic unit of financial activities—revenues and expenses. Data collection often resides in a set of individual files that must be appropriately interrelated with various data processing programs in the system. Recently designed EDP systems take advantage of a data base management system to support sophisticated data organization and manipulation. In all EDP systems, the bulk of the transactions processing is carried out on a regularly scheduled basis by specially written programs that have been designed to perform highly structured tasks.

Management Information Systems (MIS)

Most MIS include the automation of highly structured tasks among their capabilities. The major difference between MIS and EDP systems resides in the managerial orientation of its output and the degree of integration across an organization's functional areas. Both management control and operational control tasks are usually supported with the information system's output that is generally intended for middle management. This contrasts with EDP system output, which is more appropriately directed to operations personnel. The MIS support of managerial control activities has also led to much more integration of inventory, accounting, marketing, personnel, and other functional information systems than is usually found in EDP systems.

The informational focus of MIS represents a major step toward the provision of decision support. As such, MIS can contribute substantially toward planning for financial decisions. This orientation contrasts sharply with the lack of consideration of the decision-making process by many early MIS analysts and designers. Departmental expense reports that compare actual and planned expenditures, patient treatment summaries, facility staffing reports, and patient admission/ discharge transfer reports are illustrations of significant decision support activities provided under the auspices of the intelligence stage in the decision-making process. However, a budget variance report only identifies a situation requiring managerial attention. The MIS does not provide support in the design of alternative strategies to alleviate cost overruns, nor does it assist in the selection and implementation of a particular action.

Decision Support Systems (DSS)

The emergence of DSS as a distinct class of information system for management has resulted primarily from an increased emphasis on facilitating managerial decision making. Attention to decision types, levels of managerial activity, and decision-making process stages by computer-based systems designers has produced a more flexible support system. The resulting DSS has a greater capacity to handle less well structured decision situations that are more prevalent at the strategic planning and managerial control levels within an organization. A more sophisticated set of software including both a data base and a model base management system, along with an easy-to-use communication network, are available to promote active involvement by the typical manager.

DSS are especially appropriate to financial planning because their characteristics include:

- Orientation toward unstructured problems
- Availability of combinations of models and analytical techniques
- Focus on user-friendly systems in an interactive mode
- Emphasis on flexibility

These features allow nurse administrators to test a variety of different models with changing parameters. DSS are also useful in performing simulations of alternative courses of actions, especially financial impact analysis; generating optimal alternatives through the use of standardized or customized operations research techniques; and conducting sensitivity analysis to check the impact on the output of changes in input variable values.

Expert Systems (ES)

The practical application of artificial intelligence techniques to solve difficult problems in narrowly defined areas has led to the design of knowledge-based expert systems. These systems are termed knowledge-based because their performance depends upon the use of facts, beliefs, and heuristics to synthesize previously generated, problem-specific information. Expert systems are high performance computer programs that use knowledge developed in a particular domain in combination with inference mechanisms to generate results comparable to human experts. The underlying premise is that a computer system that embodies knowledge can achieve high levels of performance in task areas that, for human beings, require years of special training and education. ES are gaining in popularity and hence applicability to the financial planning area. For the moment, nurse managers should recognize that ES development must be monitored to identify opportunities for applying these systems on a more comprehensive basis in the financial management area.

Information Systems Application in Financial Planning

Since nurse administrators will be interacting with systems analysts, it becomes necessary to understand how technically oriented analysts conceive of information systems in the financial planning area. The development of useful support systems requires that nurse administrators be able to communicate their ideas about financial data availability, information requirements, and current and prospective decision-making processes to an analyst. The analyst, in turn, interprets these ideas in order to prepare a formal, precise requirements specification to guide the implementation of an information system. Clear communication to the analyst is required because of the differing perspectives of the system development participants.

The analyst is usually an intermediary who interprets the needs and requirements of the nurse administrator or other manager (person paying for development) and the user (person using the developed system) for the developer (person responsible for creating the required system). Communication and understanding are the keys to successful management systems implementation, and as much the responsibility of the nurse administrator as of the systems analyst or developer. All participants must truly understand the concepts and terminology of the system technology as well as how the application will contribute to improved financial planning.

NOTES

1. Robert A. Vraciu, "Programming, Budgeting, and Control in Health Care Organizations: The State of the Art," *Health Services Research*, Summer 1979.

2. Robert N. Anthony and David W. Young, *Management Control in Nonprofit Organizations* (Homewood, Ill.: Richard D. Irwin, Inc., 1984).

3. David W. Young, *Financial Control in Health Care* (Homewood, Ill.: Dow Jones-Irwin, 1984).

4. George A. Steiner, *Strategic Planning* (New York: Free Press, 1979).

5. Charles H. Byington, "Gross A/R: No Management Measure," *Hospital Financial Management* 33 (June 1979): 32, 34, 36.

6. Timothy Porter-O'Grady, "Financial Planning: Budgeting for Nursing, Part I," *Supervisor Nurse* 10 (August 1979): 35–37.

7. Mark A. Covaleski and Mark W. Dirsmith, "Budgeting in the Nursing Services Area: Management Control, Political, and Witchcraft Uses," *Health Care Management Review* 6 (Summer 1981): 17–24.

8. U.S. Department of Health, Education, and Welfare. *Financial Planning in Ambulatory Health Programs* (National Center for Health Services Research, DHEW Publication No. (HSM) 73–3027, pp. 17–18).

9. Timothy Porter-O'Grady, "Financial Planning: Budgeting for Nursing, Part II," *Supervisor Nurse* 10 (September 1979): 25–30.

10. Hollie Vanderzee and George Glusko, "DRGs, Variable Pricing, and Budgeting for Nursing Services," *Journal of Nursing Administration* 14 (May 1984): 11–14.

11. Charles W. Golden, Carl McDevitt, and Kenneth J. Bloch, "Good Forecasting Builds Good Budgets," *Hospital Financial Management* 35 (August 1981): 18, 19, 24–26.

12. Everette S. Gardner and Curtis P. McLaughlin, "Forecasting: A Cost Control Tool for Health Care Managers," *Health Care Management Review* 5 (Summer 1980): 31–38.

13. R. Harding Collis, "Financial Forecasts: Overcoming the Obstacles," *Hospital Financial Management* 34 (March 1980): 62–67.

14. David J. Knesper, "Financial Information Systems and the New Reimbursement Climate," *Hospital and Community Psychiatry* 35 (April 1984): 327–329.

15. R.E. Hoye and D.D. Bryant, "Current Status of Hospital Management Information System," *System Research* 1, no. 1 (1984): 55–62.

16. A.L. Eliason, *Online Business Computer Applications* (Chicago, Ill.: Science Research Associates, Inc., 1983).

17. E. Turban, "Decision Support Systems in Hospitals," *Health Care Management Review* 7, no. 3 (Summer 1982): 35–42.

18. M. Ben-Bassat, "The Role of Expert Systems in Clinical Diagnosis: A Conceptual Tutorial," *Proceedings of the Jerusalem Conference on Information Technology*, Jerusalem, Israel, 1984, pp. 632–644.

19. E.H. Shortliffe, *Computer-Based Medical Consultations: MYCIN* (New York: American Elsevier, 1976).

20. H.E. Pople, Jr., J.D. Myers, and R.A. Miller, "DIALOG: A Model of Diagnostic Logic for Internal Medicine," *Proceedings of the 4th International Conference on Artificial Intelligence*, Tbilisi, Georgia, USSR, 1975, pp. 848–855.

21. S.M. Weiss, C.A. Kulikowski, and A. Safir, "A Model-based Consultation System for the Long-term Management of Glaucoma," *Proceedings of the 5th International Conference on Artificial Intelligence*, Cambridge, Mass., 1977, pp. 826–832.

22. P. Szolovits, ed., *Artificial Intelligence in Medicine* (Boulder, Co.: Westview Press, 1982).

23. F. Hayes-Roth, D.A. Waterman, and D.B. Lenat, *Building Expert Systems* (Reading, Mass.: Addison-Wesley, 1983).

24. Rita D. Zielstorff, "Cost Effectiveness of Computerization in Nursing Practice and Administration," *Journal of Nursing Administration* 15 (February 1985): 22–26.

25. F.W. McFarlan, J.L. McKenney, and P. Pyburn, "The Information Archipelago—plotting a course," *Harvard Business Review* 61, no. 1 (January–February 1983): 145–156.

26. B. Ives and G.P. Learmonth, "The Information System as a Competitive Weapon," *Communications of the ACM* 27, no. 12 (December 1984): 1193–1201.

27. C. Wiseman, *Strategy and Computers: Information Systems as Competitive Weapons* (Homewood, Ill.: Dow Jones-Irwin, 1984).

28. Michael Porter, *Competitive Strategy* (New York: Free Press, 1980).

29. Linda Punch, "More Hospitals Turn to Software for Documenting Nursing Costs," *Modern Healthcare* 15 (June 21, 1985): 88, 91, 93.

Chapter 5

Budgeting

Budgeting is the immediate definition of a health care organization's plans. The master budget represents the articulation of specific resource allocations for a fiscal period.[1] Hence budgeting is the point at which operational plans are transformed from the abstract to the concrete. As such, there is little that is very glamorous about the budgeting task. Nonetheless it does require attention to detail and decision making before budget estimates can be finalized and resource allocation trade-offs can be made. There should be little indecision as to how much capital will be expended (i.e., determination of the capital budget), how cash flows are expected to occur during the period (i.e., determination of the cash budget), or how expenses and revenues will fluctuate (i.e., determination of the operating budget). Budgeting requires immediate attention to details.

Nurse administrators are actively involved in the budgeting process, usually at a program, work unit, or departmental level.[2] Nonetheless they should be familiar with the budgeting process as it relates to the entire organization as well as the department. By acquiring familiarity with budgeting as it fits within the organizational infrastructure, they will better understand allocation decisions that appear to suboptimize the performance of the nursing program. Such understanding is essential for translating this rationale to staff. For example, when a nursing unit is budgeted to reduce its staffing level by 1.5 full time equivalent positions, the implications may be very serious to the individual staff nurse.

A staffing reduction implies either that there is a decrease in forecasted demand for nursing services or that the nursing unit is being asked to be more productive (i.e., provide the same or more nursing services with the input of fewer nursing hours). On paper this budgeting decision or plan may not appear to be exeptionally grievous, but consider the perspective of the staff nurse. It would not be surprising to discover that staff nurses already perceive that they have been stretched to the limits of their productive capacity by the austere budget. In fact, morale might be so low that the new budget either reduces productivity (due to the cognitive

113

dissonance of the nurses and their reactive impulse to prove that they are understaffed) or instigates a high rate of turnover. Therefore, budgeting decisions must be carefully considered for their potential impact on actual operations. What might appear feasible on paper can become intolerable in reality.

When nurse administrators acquire greater familiarity with the organization's budgeting process they are better able to provide valuable input to top management about the anticipated impact on operations. They are also in a position to explain to their staff members why certain budget decisions have been made. Returning to the example of a budget reduction by the amount of 1.5 full time positions, the nurse administrator may be able to express some of the following reasons for the budget cut:

- The level of staffing in the past has been too high and now is being reduced to bring the unit on par with other nursing units.
- There is a forecasted decrease in demand for nursing services from the specific unit, and cuts are being made to balance demand with supply.
- The organization has failed to hold costs below revenues, which has resulted in deficits. All departments are participating in the budget reductions.
- The organization needs to raise the productivity of staff members. Although this means that fewer staff will be retained, remaining staff will receive higher compensation if they meet productivity goals.

There may be many other explanations for budget revisions. The nurse administrator must be able to communicate a rationale for budget reductions.

Since most health care organizations are confronting a threatening environment of prospective payment and competition, budget cuts rather than budget additions will occur more frequently in the future. For this reason, nurse administrators need to become much more sensitive to the precise influence of overall organizational operations on the nursing department. More likely than not, nurse administrators will be called on to justify why their units should continue to receive the level of budgeted funding that they had in the past. By knowing the purposes of budgets and being able to propose alternatives to the targeted cuts, the nurse administrator will function more effectively as an advocate for the nursing unit, program, or department.

BUDGET PURPOSES

Budgets represent the specific definition of broad organizational plans. As a result they have the unique capacity to represent both a planning and controlling tool. Budgets are a planning tool in the sense that they define the intentions of an organization and the allocations of resources that will help achieve these goals and objectives. Budgets are also control tools in the sense that they enable the organization to compare performance with actual resource investments. This dual capacity as planning and control instruments is beneficial to the assessment of resource investments. It permits an evaluation of the operating capacity to achieve specified targeted levels of performance while it also permits a comment on the efficiency with which those goals are achieved. When seen in this light it is apparent that budgets are valuable management tools if they are employed correctly. Recent studies of hospitals suggest that the budgeting art is improving in the application of this management tool.[3,4]

Feedforward Control on Plans

Budgets provide an essential infusion of feedforward control on organizational plans. Feedforward control is the provision of information to facilitate a manager's assessment of anticipated performance. Feedforward control is the reverse of feedback control. Feedback allows control *after* performance has occurred. Unfortunately this information comes too late to prevent dysfunctional performance or unanticipated consequences. Managers need to prevent untoward performance from happening; this is the benefit of feedforward control. Managers can anticipate problems in organizational performance. Presumably they will then be able to revise the structure or process of delivering services or producing goods to prevent the negative performance from occurring in the first place.

Nurse administrators can use this principle of feedforward control to anticipate the impact of budgets on the operations of their departments. This means that the budget should be read thoroughly to understand how budget allocations will influence operations over the coming period. In this respect the master budget is analogous to the operating manual for an automobile. It defines specific components and how they function systematically. The operating manual also provides an understanding of how the various subsystems fit together as a whole in order to provide convenient transportation. If the braking system is excessively worn, then there will be substantial ramifications for other systems in the automobile. In the same fashion the master budget facilitates understanding the specific and integrated parts or systems of a health care organization. It is then a matter of translating this reading of the master plan into a feasible interpretation for the nursing program.

Resource decisions and operating decisions will be adjusted in view of the feedforward information obtained from the master budget. This may mean revising the scheduling of nurses within various clinical units. It may imply transferring one nurse with a certain personality, or predisposition for performance, from one unit to another. It may mean implementing an extra rigorous program in supplies control in order to maintain an ample availability in every month. Alternatively there may be a need to acquire additional evidence and documentation to support a request for additional staffing. The point is that the master budget should be read for its implications for the nursing program.

Anticipating Deviations in Performance

Budgets are also valuable in anticipating deviations in performance and correcting deviations once they have been detected. Consider the following illustration of the first five months' performance of a nursing unit in a nursing home:

Month	Amount Budgeted	Actual	Variance
January	$7,800	$7,400	$ − 400
February	7,800	7,800	0
March	8,300	8,500	+ 200
April	8,300	8,600	+ 300
May	8,400	9,000	+ 600

An undesirable trend in expenditures has occurred for the nursing unit. Beginning in the shift from January to February the expenses for the nursing unit have apparently been rising. The actual expenses exceed the budgeted amount in every month after February. The projection of this trend over the entire fiscal period is not optimistic for the financial solvency of the facility.

The budget, and its comparison with actual performance, is a promising tool for management because it is possible to identify deviations in performance. It is important to determine *why* the nursing unit is above the budgeted expenditures. After identifying causal factors, some action plan must be formulated to bring expenditures back into line with reality as depicted by the master budget. In this sense, the budget has helped the nurse administrator to correct deviations from planned performance. Although the budget may not specify the precise reasons why deviations are occurring, it does facilitate investigation because it alerts the nurse administrator to deviations and it does suggest where they are occurring.

Note that effective management begins with the recognition that a problem is occurring.[5] The budget helps communicate this fact. It helps managers ascertain that performance is below (or above) planned levels before the entire fiscal period elapses. It is the responsibility of the manager to determine why the problem is present and how to rectify the situation. Hence, failure to read the budget or to chart actual performance may ultimately result in poor financial performance. The budget can only facilitate, it cannot make the decision for managers.

Establishing Performance Standards

Budgets are one of the more convenient mechanisms for establishing performance standards. This is one of the outstanding features of budgets, but it is also one of the most overlooked aspects of budgeting. This problem is endemic in management. Too often there are few standards by which to assess performance—even more often there is a failure to compare these standards with actual performance. The result is that organizations are not really managed; they are maintained. Management implies action and control. It means that a person (i.e., the manager) does something to make certain that operations produce a desired end result.

Nurse administrators recognize that health care organizations fail to manage for performance. There are many reasons for this, but the predominant reason is the retrospective payment environment inhabited by most health care organizations in the past. There was simply little reason to manage for performance. Poor performance could always be resolved simply by raising charges to increase revenues. Such attitudes and practices will now be more a memory than actual practice in view of the constraints offered by competition and prospective payment. Ultimately this change will force health care organizations to become exceptionally sensitive to performance and standard setting via budgeting.[6]

Consider the following yearly performance obtained by a nursing home from its key departments:

| Budget Area | Amount | | | % of Amount |
	Budgeted	Actual	Variance	Budgeted
Nursing	$800,000	$811,000	$ + 11,000	1.38
Dietary	240,000	195,000	− 45,000	18.75
Housekeeping	127,000	129,000	+ 2,000	1.57
Plant and Operations	150,000	155,000	+ 5,000	3.33
Social Services	13,500	12,800	− 700	5.19
Administration	48,600	48,000	− 600	1.23

How should the nursing home executive award bonuses at the end of the year? Should the nursing director receive the lowest bonus because the nursing department exceeded its budget by the highest amount ($11,000)? Should the dietary director receive the highest bonus because the department turned in a $45,000 contribution to lower expenditures? Should the director of plant and operations receive the lowest bonus because expenses for that department were proportionately higher than either nursing or housekeeping? Should the dietary director or food service manager receive a bonus that is 3 times that of the social services director and approximately 15 times that of the administrator?

The answers to these questions are not directly ascertainable from the data in the budget. But the budget does set a standard from which these questions can be asked and from which investigation can begin. This is the point of budgeting as a mechanism for standard setting. It is the basis for evaluating performance because it defines what performance is expected to be and it determines whether actual performance lived up to those expectations. Note that the term expectations is used here. The manager may know certain facts that cannot be directly expressed in figures. For example, perhaps the dietary expenses were reduced due to the alliance with a group purchasing plan that reduced food costs for the facility and due to a governmental subsidy in the form of free dairy products. Under these conditions, the dietary supervisor may not have had direct input into the favorable performance.

Nurse administrators need to envision budgets as a beginning for assessing performance. Budgets express an expectation as far as attainment of good performance. They do not provide all of the facts. Therefore when a nursing program experiences excess costs for a clearly ascertainable reason, it is the responsibility of the nurse administrator to inform the top manager or chief financial officer of the facts behind the substandard performance. In this manner the basis for accurate performance assessment is established. Nurse administrators may also use the standard to plan for future performance. Given that performance is either favorable or unfavorable according to the budget standard, new plans can be developed based on the reasons for the deviation.

Planning Cash Management

Budgets also serve the distinct purpose of helping plan for better cash management.[7] The budget is a specification of the intended performance of the organization. Hence it is also an estimate of what resources will be consumed and generated. As long as health care organizations consume resources (e.g., supplies, staff time, equipment, facilities) in the provision of services, they need to plan for sufficient cash or current assets to cover the expenses of resource consumption. The salaries and wages of staff have to be paid on a periodic basis. Supplies have to be purchased before they are consumed in order to be readily available for service delivery. Equipment is only meaningful when it is available for use. All of these resource uses mean that an organization has expended cash or other liquid assets to procure the resources.

Just as the provision of services results in consumed resources, it is also true that revenues accompany the provision of services. It is essential that these cash flows in terms of expenses and revenues be timed in such a manner that the organization is not constantly in debt or that expenses exceed revenues. The best method for controlling the cash aspects of operations is through the budgeting process. Actually the budgeting process allows a health care organization to both plan and control for cash management.

The budget reflects a forecast of when revenues will be received and when expenditures will occur. Hence the budget is a means of planning for the cash needs of an organization. Under certain conditions the organization will need to borrow cash to pay expenses, while under other conditions it will be able to set cash aside in anticipation of future expenses. Consider the seasonal fluctuations of semiannual cash needs of a nursing home over a three-year period:

Month	Variance Year 1	Variance Year 2	Variance Year 3	Average Variance
January	$ + 3,500	$ + 2,900	$ + 3,900	$ + 3,433
February	+ 1,000	+ 1,500	+ 500	+ 1,000
March	0	0	0	0
April	− 2,000	− 3,000	− 1,900	− 2,300
May	− 3,200	− 3,200	− 3,200	− 3,200
June	+ 1,600	+ 1,700	+ 1,600	+ 1,633
Total	$ + 900	$ − 100	$ + 900	$ + 566

This information provides a foundation for cash planning that should be supplemented with additional information.

Note that the nursing home begins each calendar year with a monthly cash surplus that continually erodes through March. The precise reasons for this erosion cannot be determined from the data provided, but they do suggest that the manager should attend to the causes and seek to implement a plan to use the cash to its greatest advantage (e.g., in earning interest). The cycle then shifts in March to deficits in April and May before a surplus is earned.

The fact that data for a three-year period have been gathered enables the manager to validate trends in cash needs. The manager is in the position of being able to either obtain loans to facilitate payment of debts (e.g., wages and salaries, accounts payable, or other current and long-term obligations) or plan a savings program to prevent borrowing. There is no guarantee that the fourth year in the nursing home's performance will result in the same cash needs as those for the first three years; however the trends should be repeated unless there has been some unusual change that may alter the cash flow.

OVERVIEW OF THE BUDGET PROCESS

Nurse administrators need to understand the specific steps involved in the budgeting process.[8] These steps include:

1. Develop assumptions and prepare projections on estimated demand and use—the statistical forecast.
2. Prepare expense forecasts.
3. Prepare a capital budget.
4. Prepare revenue forecasts.
5. Prepare a budgeted income statement.

6. Adjust charges and budgets as necessary.
7. Develop a cash budget.

Note that these steps may not always be followed in the order that they are presented above. Furthermore, some of the steps may be deleted entirely, depending on the situation. These steps are only illustrative, but most health care organizations and programs will use these or similar steps in their budgeting process.[9]

Nurse administrators need to be familiar with the budget process, yet they should not become so oriented to one system or another that they cannot adapt to a different process. It is essential that the core elements of budgeting be understood. In this regard three main components of the master budget should be calculated.[10] The operating budget is the primary element of the annual budget. It incorporates estimates of utilization, expenses, and revenues. In the budgeting process outlined above it is apparent that the operating budget is the beginning point for the master budget.

The capital budget presents a forecast of expenditures on assets such as plant and equipment. The capital budget therefore is actually a form of expense budget but is usually listed separately because it involves investments in capital assets, not operating expenses. The capital budget is considered here after the expense forecast to underscore the similarity between these estimates. The third main component of the annual budget is the cash budget. It presents an estimate of cash receipts and disbursements. The cash budget is formulated to prepare contingency plans for acquiring cash to be used in covering current operations. At points it may be necessary to obtain short-term loans in order to manage cash flows.

The Statistical Forecast

The forecast of use or the statistical forecast is the fundamental planning document for a health care organization. It is the basis upon which all budgets are formulated and hence it has critical importance for the financial solvency of health care organizations. If the forecast is incorrect, then the remainder of the budgeting process will also be incorrect. It is very difficult to arrive at a precise estimate of use because there are many factors that affect demand. This inability to attain precision is usually managed by developing several projections.

For example, a nursing administrator might estimate high and low demand, or high, medium, and low demand. Then separate budgets are created around these estimates. Another method is to use flexible budgeting that permits timely adjustments in the master budget as variables change. Whatever method is used, recognize that forecasting is an imprecise science.

In illustrating the budgeting process, it is convenient to consider the case of Moraine Hospital, a 50-bed acute care hospital serving a rural population in the

Rocky Mountain states. As a rural hospital, it has experienced some fluctuations in demand for its services in the past. Currently the beds are allocated to three service areas:

General-Surgical	35
Intensive Care	10
Obstetrics	5
Total	50

For these 50 beds, the number of patient days served now totals 16,425, or a 90 percent occupancy rate. This is an exceptional level of occupancy for a general rural hospital. Part of the success must be attributed to the administrator, who has gone to great lengths to involve the local medical staff and to develop a network in surrounding communities.

The immediate problem facing Moraine Hospital is the planned construction of a new 100-bed hospital in a community 45 miles away. Although serving a different catchment area, this hospital may influence the occupancy and admissions at Moraine Hospital. Furthermore, this impact is admittedly very likely because an investor-owned chain of hospitals will be constructing the facility. Therefore it is probable that the new hospital will rely upon extensive investments in marketing in order to maintain a viable level of occupancy. This complicates the fact that Moraine Hospital has always had an explicit policy of low room rates. This policy is part of the voluntary orientation of Moraine Hospital and has been designed to prevent local physicians from referring patients to urban tertiary care centers.

Moraine must reassess its charges and budgets this year in view of the planned construction of the new competitive hospital. At most, Moraine has two years to adjust its rates before the new hospital is operating. The purpose of any proposed rate increase is to better reflect the costs of providing care. It also creates a retained surplus that will be necessary to promote Moraine Hospital's services when its new competition is operating. Clearly Moraine Hospital is facing a major budgeting crisis. The budget must reflect the changed environment, yet it must also address the policies and standard operating procedures of the past.

The first step in budgeting for Moraine Hospital is to create a statistical forecast. With existing records it is possible to define the use that Moraine experienced last year. What is more difficult is to estimate changes in use—there are few reliable guides that Moraine Hospital can adopt for estimating use in the future. Feasible techniques include:

- estimating increases by trend analysis (i.e., determining growth rates in use areas according to prior years' performance)
- estimating increases by informed opinion (i.e., forecasts suggested by the administrative staff according to their intuition and expertise)[11]

- analyzing demographics, epidemiology, and practice patterns by sophisticated quantitative methods

For this situation, it is assumed that the administration of Moraine Hospital has estimated the increases/decreases of use.

A representative statistical forecast might include the following elements that represent the basis for the master budget:

		Forecast of Use	
	Last Year	Forecasted Increase (%)	Budgeted
Admissions			
General-Surgical	1,679	3	1,729
Intensive Care	339	1	342
Obstetrics	256	2	261
Patient Days (Occupancy) General-Surgical			
(92%)	11,753	1	11,871
Intensive Care			
(93%)	3,394	2	3,462
Obstetrics (70%)	1,278	2	1,304
Support Services			
Laboratory Tests	3,411	12	3,820
X-rays	2,877	10	3,165
Drug Prescriptions Dispensed	3,000	13	3,390
Surgical Procedures	1,700	2	1,734
Obstetrical Procedures	500	2	510

Note that the statistical forecast is the best estimate on the part of Moraine Hospital about use in the coming year. Last year's figures are derived from the hospital's records. The forecasted increase is determined by the administrator through experience, intuition, and assessment of the forthcoming changes. The budgeted use column simply represents last year's statistics increased by the forecasted additional amount (e.g., for general-surgical: 1,679 admissions $\times$ 1.03 = 1,729 admissions).

Expense Forecast

The second step in the budgeting process is to estimate the expenses that will be incurred given anticipated increases in use and in prices. Here again the health care manager is often confronted by less than perfect information. As a result it is often necessary to guess the increases. Such an estimate need not be an uninformed guess. It is possible to assess the variables that might influence increases in expenses, including general inflation in the economy, historical price increases from suppliers, advance notices of price increases from suppliers, use, or other fairly reliable sources of information.[12]

A key factor in deriving accurate estimates of expenses is to involve department and program heads.[13] These managers are very familiar with trends in expenses relating to their specific areas. For example, nursing administrators will need to estimate the impact of staffing expenses on the nursing department budget.[14] By using nursing pools within the facility, it may be possible to reduce expenditures on nursing staff. In other situations, external nursing pools or registries will be used to minimize the fixed costs associated with nursing staff. These staffing variations will be directly influenced by changes in average daily census and average occupancy.

Moraine Hospital will break down its expenses into three categories: revenue adjustment; supplies; and salaries, wages, and professional fees. It is important to recognize that these three categories are not the only meaningful breakdown of expenses that a health care organization will necessarily have. There may be more or fewer depending on the complexity of the organization, its accounts, and its personnel or related professional staff.

Expense Forecast

	Last Year	Forecasted Increases (%)	Budgeted
Revenue Adjustments			
Bad Debts	$ 15,200	10	$ 16,720
Contractual			
Allowances	30,759	10	33,835
Charitable Care	17,673	5	18,557
	63,632		69,112
Supplies			
General-Surgical	112,000	5	117,600
Intensive Care	53,000	3	54,590
Obstetrics	9,000	4	9,360
Laboratory	49,000	16	56,840
Radiology	51,000	17	59,670
Pharmacy	107,000	15	123,050
Food Service	122,000	7	130,540
Housekeeping	17,689	6	18,750
Medical Records	4,110	5	4,356
Administration	72,000	7	77,040
	596,799		651,796

Salaries, Wages, and Professional Fees			
Radiology	82,000	2	83,640
Nursing	720,000	2	734,400
Laboratory	59,000	2	60,180
Pharmacy	48,000	2	48,960
Food Service	200,000	2	204,000
Housekeeping	230,000	2	234,600
Medical Records	112,000	2	114,240
Administration	98,000	2	99,960
	1,549,000		1,579,980

As with the statistical forecast, there is no guarantee that any of the forecasted adjustments will actually happen. Here is where the importance of preparing multiple budgets on the basis of alternative estimates enters into the manager's budgeting process. Clearly the creation of multiple budgets suggests that more time will have to be allocated to budgeting, but the only alternative is to place confidence in a single forecast. Often a financial officer will identify only those items that are most susceptible to variation and then formulate several budgets. This approach reduces the amount of time devoted to recalculating the alternative budget.

Nurse administrators should recognize that technology is increasingly available to minimize the effort at refiguring budgets on the basis of new premises and forecasts. The advent of computerized information systems and decision support systems are the leading examples of this technology. Moreover, proliferating personal computers have the necessary core capacity to run basic budgeting estimates. Software is readily available to facilitate variable budgeting. Not every nurse administrator will have such technology available, but it is critical to be aware that such management aids are available for situations where computations are lengthy or where changes are consistently entered into accounts.

Capital Requests Budget

The third step in the budgeting process for Moraine Hospital is to estimate all expenditures for plant and equipment. Usually a separate committee of the board of directors and management staff such as the finance committee is responsible for formulating the budget. The reason that the capital budget is created at the top management level relates to the sources of requests. In Moraine Hospital's case, like other hospitals, many requests will come from the medical staff. These requests will often be very expensive and may alter the basic services of the overall organization. In other words, it is probable that the capital budget will necessitate strategic-level decisions. Top management will be responsible for analyzing these requests and preparing appropriate documentation for the board of directors.

Nurse administrators will probably participate in capital budgeting from the perspective of the equipment requests within nursing services. They will need to justify equipment requests on the basis of use. This justification typically is presented to the finance committee because not every capital budget request is guaranteed of being funded. In more advanced health care organizations, every budget item must be justified before funding. However, in many cases medical staff requests are not accompanied by appropriate documentation. The medical staff have political power that permits their requests to be funded even though they lack documentation or justification. These practices are changing because the restrictions of prospective payment and competition are forcing health care organizations to use more financial discretion in capital asset requests. The increasingly prevalent criterion used in determining capital requests is the return on investment possible from a piece of equipment or other capital asset.

Nurse administrators may also participate in capital budgeting in terms of projecting clinical support required for new technological acquisitions or for new programs. In these situations the nurse administrator must estimate the extent to which nursing services will use the equipment or program services. This estimate is then aggregated with other possible use estimates in arriving at a logical projection of need for new equipment or services.

In the case of Moraine Hospital, assume that the following capital budget was approved by the finance committee. The items preceded by an asterisk represent expenditures that are approved only if there is an operating surplus; all other items were viewed as essential capital expenditures:

Capital Budget Requests

Plant	High Priority	Low Priority
Replacement of Roof on East Wing	$ 79,000	
*Sinking Fund for Future Replacement of Roof on West Wing		85,000
*Expansion of Physicians' Parking Lot		125,000
*Construction of Medical Office Building		717,000
Equipment		
2 Therapeutic Tubs	4,918	
Cardiac Care Equipment	10,716	
Assorted Laboratory Equipment	3,987	
Assorted Nursing Equipment	4,745	
*Assorted Housekeeping Equipment		2,999
*Portable Radiology Equipment		8,113
TOTAL	$103,366	$938,112

Two budget figures are calculated. The first is the plant and equipment expenditures that have highest priority for the hospital. The second figure represents expenditures that are desired but not necessary in the forthcoming year.

One capital expense that is not presented in the capital budget requests is the existing interest payment on the loan for the facilities at Moraine Hospital. These expenses related to capital assets are investments that already have been made; hence it is inappropriate to incorporate this cost in the capital requests budget. A better alternative is to include interest payments on capital assets in the expense budget, or in a separate budget devoted to items that are not easily classified as operating expenses.

In order to present a complete profile of expenses for Moraine Hospital we will assume that its interest expenses are $125,000 per year. There is sufficient justification for not including this in the capital budget requests above because the expenditure has already been made. On the other hand, it is inappropriate to include this as an operating expense because it is not an expense associated with services. It is an asset-related expense. A common convention is to view interest expense as the cost of doing business each year. Unless the hospital makes an expenditure on plant, there will be no facility in which to house the services. The important concern is to integrate the cost of long-term assets within one of the budgets—operating expense, capital requests, or a separate budget for capital expenses.

Another expense that is not normally included with operating expenses is depreciation. Remember that the depreciation expense accounts for the deterioration of plant and equipment and as such it is not an out-of-pocket expense. In other words, an organization does not have to make cash payments to cover this expense, although in concept it pays through the use of the assets. Depreciation expenses are not normally included in the operating budget because like interest expenses they represent a long-run expense for (basically) fixed assets. Consequently, both depreciation expenses and interest expenses are conveniently managed by incorporating them in the income statement.

In the capital requests budget illustrated above it is apparent that the finance committee used a conservative approach to approving expenditures or assets. The essential capital requests budget is $103,366, while an additional $938,112 in expenditures has been approved if funds become available. It is this commitment to prioritizing capital expenditures that can facilitate the budgeting process. Moraine Hospital could go one step further by ranking each essential and desired capital asset (i.e., requests with an asterisk). In this manner the administrator would be able to approve the purchase of the assets as revenues permitted, rather than wait for approval first from the finance committee.

Revenue Forecast

Once all expenses have been budgeted, it is appropriate to estimate revenues that will be earned. As with the forecasts for expense items, the revenue forecast depends extensively on the statistical utilization estimates. The need for accuracy in the statistical forecast is apparent at this point. Since virtually all budgets are related to estimates of use, it is vital to prevent multiplied errors by formulating reliable estimates at the beginning of the budgeting process.

The revenue forecast for Moraine Hospital can be calculated using past room rates and charges. Unless a decision has already been made on rates and charges for the coming year, it is inappropriate to estimate what the rates and charges should be. The precise determination of new rates comes after the projected revenues at existing rates have been compared with the expense budgets. The rationale for this approach is simple. There may be no reason to change a rate or room charge because the pricing structure already provides for net income. Alternatively, it is possible that only a few of the room rates or service charges should be altered in order to break even (or attain other financial goals). This approach offers a rationale for which rates and charges are changed. Otherwise, the manager is merely using the assumption that rates have to be adjusted. There should be some inherent logic behind the rate changes.

The calculation of anticipated revenues for health care organizations such as Moraine Hospital is becoming increasingly complex as third party payers develop more sophisticated payment practices. For example, hospitals formerly were paid on a per diem basis. However, Medicare's introduction of diagnosis related group reimbursement uses patient admissions as the standard unit of payment. Other prospective payment plans are based on capitated prepayment. Presently, there is no single, universal payment mechanism because not all insurers are prepared to follow the Medicare model. Admittedly, some states have adopted all-payer plans that legislate payment per admission. However, there still is great diversity in payment plans nationwide. Even if a universal payment plan centered on admissions were adopted in the near future, it would be only transitory. Projections suggest that vouchers or capitated prepayment will replace the Medicare admission-oriented plan.

In view of the ambiguity in payment patterns, it is impossible to conclude that one particular system will confront nurses in their financial management responsibilities. We recommend that nurses carefully monitor the reimbursement trends within their own state and the prevalent third parties funding health care for their patients. In this manner, it will be possible to adjust the budgeting process and other financial management functions to the structure and incentives offered in new third party reimbursement plans.

Meanwhile, it is assumed that Moraine Hospital inhabits a payment environment that is essentially a per diem context. Moraine Hospital is anticipating the following revenues using the old room rate and charge schedule:

Forecast of Revenues

	Existing Rate	Revenue Last Year	Projected Revenue
Patient Care Revenues*			
General-Surgical	$115.00	$1,351,595	$1,365,165
Intensive Care	156.00	529,464	540,072
Obstetrics	109.00	139,302	142,136
Support Services Revenues**			
Laboratory Tests	$ 12.50	42,638	47,750
X-rays	43.00	123,711	136,095
Drug Prescriptions	13.00	39,000	44,070
Surgical Procedures	35.00	59,500	60,690
Obstetrical Procedures	47.00	23,500	23,970
TOTAL		$2,308,710	$2,359,948

* = Charge per patient day
** = Charge per patient treated

It is important to note that the existing rate for the patient care revenues represents a charge per patient day. In order to determine the amount of revenue generated for each clinical area, it is necessary to multiply the charge per patient day by the number of patient days delivered last year, and by the forecasted number of patient days to be delivered. For example, last year the general-surgical service provided 11,753 days of inpatient care and is forecasted to provide 11,871 days of inpatient care. The revenue for last year is calculated as $115 × 11,753 = $1,351,595; projected revenue for next year is calculated as $115 × 11,871 = $1,365,165. The other clinical areas are also calculated using past and forecasted patient days served per year, multiplied by the room charge.

It is also appropriate to speak in terms of estimated revenue because there is a possibility that the hospital will not collect the entire charge. There may be discounts, contractual allowances, bad debts, or charity care provided.[15] In these cases the entire charge is not collected, and in some instances no revenues are collected. These adjustments to income can be resolved under the income statement. The point is that gross accounts receivable are receivable only until they are collected.[16,17]

The rate for support services is a charge per patient treated. Therefore each patient or case receiving support services will be charged a specific amount according to a rate schedule. To determine the potential revenue derived from providing these services it is necessary to multiply the support service charge by the number of services or procedures performed. For example, there were 3,411 laboratory tests performed last year by Moraine Hospital, and it is anticipated that 3,820 laboratory tests will be performed in the coming year. This will result in charges respectively of $42,638 (i.e., $12.50 × 3,411 = $42,638) for last year and $47,750 (i.e., 3,820 × $12.50 = $47,750) for the coming year. The remaining support services and procedures are calculated in the same fashion.

It is apparent from the forecast of revenues that projected revenues are $2,359,948 for the forthcoming year. This is $51,238 (i.e., $2,359,948 − $2,308,710 = $51,238) more than the preceding year. The question is whether this revenue is sufficient to cover all expenses or whether rates will have to be raised. By calculating the revenues at the existing rate, a convenient comparison with the prior year's performance can be made. This is undoubtedly valuable information that would otherwise be lost if the hospital had decided to revise its rates a priori.

Income Statement

Moraine Hospital is now in the position of being able to calculate an income statement. It has all of the essential ingredients calculated in the budgets—operating expenses, capital budget, and revenue forecasts. The hospital must now determine its solvency:

Income Statement

	Last Year	Projected Next Year
Revenues		
Patient Care	$2,020,361	$2,047,373
Support Services	288,349	312,575
TOTAL	2,308,710	2,359,948
Expenses		
Supplies	596,799	651,796
Salaries, Wages, and Professional Fees	1,549,000	1,579,980
TOTAL	2,145,799	2,231,776
Net Before Adjustments	162,911	128,172
Revenue Adjustments	63,632	69,112
Less Interest Expense	125,000	125,000
Net Before Depreciation	(25,721)	(65,940)
Depreciation Expense	75,000	75,000
Net Income	$ (100,721)	$ (140,940)

The pro forma income statement for Moraine Hospital suggests that its fiscal solvency is in jeopardy. Both the current and projected income statements suggest that Moraine Hospital is losing money, and the losses are higher in the forthcoming year. The net income before depreciation is − $25,721 in the past year and − $65,940 for next year. These results suggest that one of two things may be happening at Moraine Hospital. Either expenses are too high or revenues are too low. From the description of Moraine Hospital, it is more likely that revenues are too low. The policy of Moraine has been to maintain low charges in order to provide a community orientation. However, the future environment is threatening the long-run viability of this policy. If nothing else, the financial constraints from losses during the last year jeopardize the ability to maintain such a policy in the coming year.

Adjusting Charges

Clearly the problem before Moraine Hospital is to determine how much to raise room rates and charges. This process of adjusting prices can be undertaken either analytically or through estimations by the management staff. The so-called analytical approach relies on economic techniques to calculate prices. Unfortunately, these techniques are influenced by the differential prices charged to patients and third party payers. Various contractual discounts, allowances, and adjustments effectively reduce the precision of the calculations, and other external considerations must be considered. The mission of a hospital, and its board members' values, will often militate the quantitative calculation of rates. The growth of competition is another factor that can adversely affect the precise setting of rates.

Rate setting is also affected by the type of reimbursement methods used by third party payers. With the trend toward prospective payment, hospitals are discovering that they have little actual input into third party rate determination. This is currently true for Medicare, where rates are predetermined and a per admission basis is used. Increasingly, it is a matter of maintaining good accounting records to justify payment beyond these predetermined admission rates for patients who require intense care. As payment systems gravitate toward capitated plans, the importance of cost estimations in establishing a financially feasible capitated rate will increase.

Most of these factors that disturb the precision of quantitatively determining rates are operating for Moraine Hospital. A new hospital is scheduled to be built in a nearby community in two years. The hospital has maintained a strong community focus and is unlikely to revise this orientation in the future. Greater marketing is needed. When all of these factors are added together it is apparent that Moraine Hospital will need to be very careful in determining its rates. For purposes of illustration, it is possible to observe in the adjusted income statement the impact from a 6 percent average charge increase. Note that the net income loss in the past year is approximately 5 percent of total revenues, while the projected loss is approximately 6 percent (i.e., $140,940 ÷ $2,359,948 = .06) of total revenues in the next year's budget.

The issue is whether a 6 percent increase in rates will cover the forecasted expenses. Also, why was a figure of 5.9 not chosen, or a figure of 7.4? Why should 6 percent be the factor for raising rates? There are two good reasons. First, the 6 percent figure was ascertained from the percentage of revenue deficit. It was analytically determined—there is a clear rationale for choosing this rate increase in order to balance expenses and revenue. Second, the 6 percent figure is within tolerable limits for the hospital. Note that many of the forecasted use increases were in the range of 2.3 percent. Price increases for supplies varied from 0 to 7 percent. Although 6 percent is high considering these ranges, it is not so high that it is unreasonable. But more importantly, Moraine Hospital must attain financial solvency. That is the bottom line.

Adjusted Income Statement

	Last Year	Next Year
Adjusted Revenues (+6%)	$2,447,233	$2,501,545
Expenses	2,145,799	2,231,776
Net Before Adjustments	301,434	269,769
Adjustments and Interest	188,632	194,112
Net Before Depreciation	112,802	75,657
Depreciation Expenses	75,000	75,000
Net Income	$ 37,802	$ 657

The increase of room rates and charges by an average 6 percent has resolved the financial solvency issue for Moraine Hospital. It is now virtually breaking even in the forthcoming year. Meanwhile, if it had adjusted its rates upward by 6 percent in the last year it would have maintained a positive operating surplus.

Caution should be used in assessing the projected income statements. As was previously mentioned, depreciation expense is not truly an out-of-pocket expense. Therefore Moraine Hospital has some flexibility in the amount of approximately $75,000. It is feasible that the hospital could forgo a rate increase, but in order to make a full determination it would be necessary to examine the balance sheet to assess the full financial profits of the hospital.

Note also that no increase in revenue adjustments is assumed. This may be a tenuous premise because not every dollar of higher revenue will be received.

Readjustments in contractual allowances and higher bad debts would undoubtedly raise this figure. For the illustration, however, the figure has been kept constant.

Even though an average 6 percent rate increase has been prescribed, there still is an issue about how that increase will be distributed. Will the increase be uniformly applied? Or will the general-surgical rates receive a higher increase compared with the obstetrics and intensive care services? The room rate and charge adjustments could be managed in several ways:

- A uniform percentage increase could be applied to all revenue-generating centers and then adjusted within each center on the basis of use (e.g., per patient day, per case, etc.).
- A differential percentage increase could be applied to the revenue-generating centers (e.g. 75 percent of needed additional revenues to patient care and 25 percent of additional revenues to support services).
- Differential increases could be applied in the specific components of the revenue centers (e.g., general-surgical and intensive care may receive increases while obstetrics is kept at existing rates in order to maintain demand for the obstetrics unit and to reinforce commitment to the obstetrics area with a new competitor moving in).
- Differential increases could be applied on the basis of added cost (i.e., increases would be allocated to the respective increases in costs in the specific service areas).

There are other viable methods of determining rate increases. It is vital that health care organizations adopt a rationale for their cost increases that is tied in some manner directly to the factors that make costs vary. Across-the-board percentage increases are merely a convention to circumvent analysis and logical thinking about how rate changes should be instituted.

Third party payers have been progressively adopting the position that charges must be justified through costs. Therefore a health care organization must be able to accurately document its cost experience and in so doing provide evidence that a rate adjustment is legitimate. Reimbursers are rapidly evolving to the point that changes in rates will be allowed only when costs demand an increase. Therefore health care providers must be very careful to gather and record cost data that validate their requests. For example, Moraine Hospital must carefully document both use *and* price increases in order to make a strong case for a rate change. Furthermore, Moraine Hospital should be able to explain why it has chosen a differential pricing strategy for the patient care and support service revenues.

Developing a Cash Budget

A final step in the budgeting process is to develop a cash budget. The purpose of the cash budget is to ascertain whether short-term loans will have to be secured in order to cover the cost of operations. There are several methods of planning for cash needs. One approach charts the respective receipts and disbursements over the entire fiscal period (e.g., one year). This method recognizes that there are inherent fluctuations in cash management that cannot be controlled from month to month. This variability is tolerated by building a cash reserve to manage the fluctuations. Short-term loans are pursued only in exceptional circumstances. Since short-term financing is very expensive, any health care organization wants to avoid these expenses.

Another prevalent approach to planning cash needs is to break down the budget into monthly (or similar) operating periods. Moraine Hospital would need to determine monthly use and monthly expenses in order to plan its cash needs across twelve periods. The obvious advantage of using this approach is that it helps avoid unnecessary short-term borrowing if it can be ascertained when cash needs are likely to exceed reserves. For example, if July is the month in which accounts receivable tend to lag and when expenditures are high (due to taking advantage of trade credits and discounts in previous months), the hospital may be able to enforce additional savings to build a reserve for this high cash demand, thereby avoiding the costs of short-term borrowing.

Since the use and expense data for Moraine Hospital are not broken down on a monthly basis, it is appropriate to forecast a yearly cash budget using an assumption that the hospital has $65,000 in cash reserves (i.e., in demand deposits and 90-day certificates of deposit that will mature before the next calendar fiscal period begins). Assume that the 6 percent across the board rate increase prevails in charges.

Cash Budget

Cash on Hand (beginning of year)		
Demand Deposits and Certificates of Deposit		$ 65,000
Accounts Receivable		
Patient Care	$2,170,215	
Support Services	331,330	
		2,501,545
		2,566,545
Expenses		
Supplies	651,796	
Salaries, Wages, and Professional Fees	1,579,980	
		2,231,776
		334,769
Other Expenses		
Revenue Adjustments	69,112	
Interest Expense	125,000	
		194,112
		140,657

Net Funds
Capital Expenditures
    Roof—East Wing   79,000
    Equipment   24,366
                                                                    103,366
    Net Cash on Hand (end of year) $ 37,291

The cash budget indicates that with a six percent rate increase Moraine Hospital will have $37,291 on hand at the end of the year. The yearly performance assumes that the highest priority capital asset expenditures on roof and equipment will be made. Therefore, even with the rate increase, Moraine Hospital is driving down its cash reserves by $27,709 (i.e., $65,000 − $37,291 = $27,709). This is probably unacceptable to the management of the hospital because of future capital needs. There is also a problem with the changing environment. Hence it is likely that Moraine Hospital will have to raise its rates in order to prepare for the future.

Summary of the Budgeting Process

Even though the preceding analysis has focused on an organization's budgeting process, it is essential to realize that many of the same steps and thought processes must be employed to formulate an accurate program or department budget. The level of detail will be more critical. The organization's records are founded upon aggregations at the departmental and program levels. The point is that specific accounts, expenses, use, productivity, and forecasting methods may vary, but the process remains the same.

PREPARING THE DEPARTMENTAL BUDGET

Conceptually, a departmental budget follows the same steps identified for an organization such as Moraine Hospital. However, the primary difference between an organizational and departmental budget relates to the level of specificity. The departmental budget is the fundamental information base from which the overall budget is calculated. Hence, it is very detailed and requires very accurate determination of use and costs in order to be valuable as a management tool. In view of this specificity, it is critical that directors of nursing services and head nurses participate actively in the budgeting process. They must eventually translate the plan for action specificed in the budget into actual services. Additionally, they are often able to provide explanations regarding past budget variances and anticipated problems that might prevent attainment of projected budget goals.

Steps in the Budgeting Process

The precise steps completed at the department head and head nurse levels are partially influenced by the extent to which an organization is using a bottom-up or top-down approach to budget formation. A top-down approach is essentially a centralized effort that is completed by the budget director or a similar financial/ accounting representative. Typically, the chief financial officer delegates preparation of the budget to financial staff personnel. They acquire projections of utilization and establish preliminary budgets for specific departments with projected staffing patterns (usually based on historical trends). Under the top-down approach the nursing administrator is relieved of much of the burden in calculating pro forma budgets. However, this approach also minimizes the control of the nursing department over the determination of estimates and required funding. In essence, control is retained by top management.

An increasingly prevalent budgeting approach is to decentralize the entire process. Under this methodology the director of nursing, administrative assistants, and head nurses have much more responsibility. They may collect information on utilization trends and forecasts of service units from departmental or organizational data bases. They may work with financial, accounting, or data processing staff in retrieving these data if they are contained in a computerized information system. Additionally, they acquire personnel data, specifically staff hours and expenses, to estimate staffing levels and expenses. In sum, the bottom-up approach leaves the budgeting process to specific departments for the initial or pro forma calculations. The budgeting director may provide staff to assist in various phases, but the primary responsibility is delegated downward. Once these departmental efforts have been completed, they are integrated by the budget director. After this point, there are successive refinements of the budget through negotiations with specific departments.

Given the increasing pressure in the health care environment for cost control, it is probable that a decentralized format will become more prevalent in health care organizations. The nursing budget is commonly a significant proportion of the total budget. The nursing administrative staff will become active participants in forecasting staffing levels given the pressures to hold down costs. They must be able to translate these pressures into anticipated changes in staffing including overall coverage, nursing hours per patient day, and indirect care. Second, they will be responsible for interpreting the proposed budget for the nursing team. Clearly, the nursing department will be very involved in budgeting even if other departments have a less active role. In view of this trend, it is vital that nurse administrators familiarize themselves with the steps in the budgeting process to become the best representatives and advocates for nursing services.

A detailed model of the planning and budgeting process for nursing services is presented in Figure 5–1. According to this model there are eight key steps

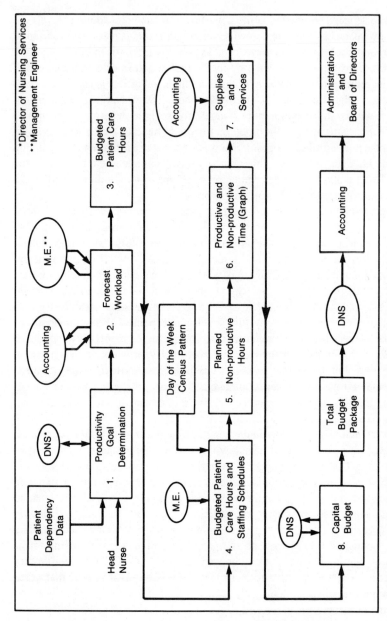

Figure 5–1 The Planning and Budgeting Process for Nursing Services

Source: Reprinted from *Journal of Nursing Administration*, Vol. 12, p. 16, with permission of J.B. Lippincott Company, © May 1982.

involved in formulating a budget for the nursing department. Each step of this model builds upon previous steps as well as information supplied from organizational records. In several steps the actual involvement of staff from nursing, finance, accounting, and management engineering is needed to facilitate documentation or calculation of pertinent cost and use patterns.

The primary ingredient in a nursing department budget is the specified level of funding for staffing. As with the overall budgeting process, the staffing plan is based on the best estimates of future demand. Generally, these estimates are largely if not entirely based on prior performance. For example, Step 1 in Figure 5–1 indicates that the nursing department must project its productivity goals. Productivity is defined as a ratio of output to input. The higher the productivity, the higher the amount of nursing services delivered for the input of resources (i.e., staff time). In order to be effective, productivity goals should be specified at the beginning of the budgeting process. They set a standard throughout the year for effort from the staff. They also influence the final budget estimates for labor required (i.e., nursing hours) and hence projected expenses for nursing services.

Step 2 in Figure 5–1 indicates that the workload for the nursing department is estimated with the assistance of the accounting (or fiscal services) department and in some instances management engineers (i.e., analysts who study specific aspects of operations such as patient loads within a nursing unit on a weekly or monthly basis). The purpose of this step is to project the patient days that will be provided in a specific nursing unit and correlate them with a preferred staffing level. Step 3 is a derivative of Step 2. Here the patient care hours are projected relative to the preferred staffing level (i.e., number of full time equivalent nurses). These patient care hour projections must acknowledge the variations in nursing care intensity between shifts (e.g., days, evenings, and nights). Step 2 and Step 3 are illustrated in Table 5–1.

Table 5–1 presents the projected patient census for Step 2 on a monthly basis for a specific nursing unit. These data have been obtained from historical utilization data and adjusted for estimated changes in demand. The nursing director or head nurse for this unit should verify the validity of these projections. The projections in Step 2 serve as a basis for preliminary planning of a monthly staffing schedule in June. As Table 5–1 indicates, the number of nursing days (eight-hour shifts) is calculated for each week. These weekly totals must then be allocated to specific shifts such as days, evenings, or nights. The intensity of staffing may vary among shifts. For example, the day and evening shifts are each allocated 40 percent of the nursing days while the night shift receives a 20 percent allocation. On the basis of these data, it is possible to proceed to Step 4 in Figure 5–1 where patient care hours and staffing schedules are further decomposed to produce a weekly staffing schedule.

Step 5 in the budgeting process incorporates planned nonproductive time allocations for nurses. Allowances are made for vacation and holiday time,

Table 5–1 Staffing Projections in a Nursing Unit

Month	Patient Census Projected from Historical Records
January	700 patient days
February	800
•	•
•	•
•	•
June	815
•	•
•	•
•	•
November	580
December	570

Staffing Schedule for June

Week	Census	Nursing Hours per Patient Day	Total Nursing Hours per Week	Number of Nursing Days (8-Hour Shifts)
1	210	3.5	735.0	91.9
2	200	3.5	700.0	87.5
3	205	3.5	717.5	89.7
4	200	3.5	735.0	91.9
Total	815			

overtime devoted to nursing activities, administrative time, and other assignments (e.g., attendance at continuing education seminars). The culmination of the five steps is a labor budget that reflects both productive and nonproductive time. Such a budget can be depicted visually as shown in Figure 5–2. This is Step 6 in the budgeting process.

Step 7 in Figure 5–1 involves the calculation of supplies and services expenses. These data, typically obtained from accounting records, include the cost of supplies, contracts for services (e.g., management, physician services, and equipment maintenance), pharmaceuticals, and overhead, among other expenses. Finally, in Step 8 the director of nursing prepares the capital budget for new equipment or the replacement of equipment. The culmination of Step 1 to Step 8 is the formulation of the total budget. The director of nursing (in this model) then negotiates this budget with the accounting or finance department before it is presented to top management and the board of directors for approval.

BUDGET TIMETABLE

Nurse administrators should be familiar with budget timetables. Such timetables vary considerably from organization to organization, and from department

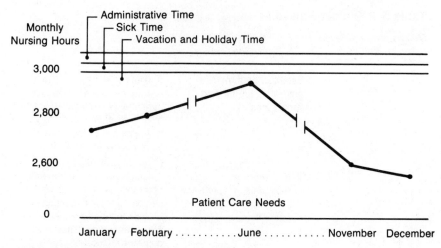

Figure 5–2 Staff Planning Graph

Source: Adapted from *Journal of Nursing Administration*, Vol. 12, p. 37, with permission of J.B. Lippincott Company, © June 1982.

to department; however, the key is to plan specific milestones and activities. In this fashion there is a structure to guide the budgeting process. Table 5–2 is an example of a budget timetable for Moraine Hospital. The key in the budget timetable is to allow plenty of time. Time is needed to gather and analyze data, to anticipate and resolve deficiencies, and to allow the process to run its natural course.

FLEXIBLE BUDGETING

Nurse administrators will encounter a form of budgeting that is becoming increasingly prevalent due to the availability of computer systems.[18] Health care institutions are turning to flexible budgeting to address variances in monthly volume and utilization (or from one performance period to the next).[19] The budgeting process described in this chapter represents a static or unchanging budget; that is, a master budget that is formulated around one level (or a very limited number of levels) of estimated demand. The problem with such a budget is fairly evident. It does not account for alterations in expenses, revenues, or volume. Since the complex environment of the health care organization is ever-changing, and since rather major changes are instituted by third party payers in any given fiscal period, it is vital to adapt a budget to these changes.

Flexible budgeting is centered around various levels of utilization and requires an understanding of cost behavior:[20–24]

Table 5–2 Budget Timetable

Months before Initiation of Budget	Goal	Activity
6	Establish performance guidelines for the next fiscal period	Budget committee meets and reviews past fiscal period performance. Committee sets guidelines after analyzing forecasts and estimates from the planning and financial staff.
5	Communicate guidelines to managers of departments and programs	Chief financial officer meets with the managers of departments, programs, or other budget centers to explain the guidelines for forthcoming fiscal period, concentrating on rationale for guidelines. Questions are clarified.
4	Submit proposed budgets for each unit	Managers take the guidelines and apply them to the operations of their specific units. They note deviances and gather documentation for justifying added expenditures that violate the guidelines.
3	Formulate a comprehensive pro forma budget	Chief financial officer reviews the proposed budgets and seeks clarification from specific managers.
2	Review the pro forma budget	Budget committee meets with managers to hear their input on the proposed budget.
1	Modify and approve the budget	Budget committee adjusts the budget as needed and disseminates the budget to managers.
0	Adhere to budget in operations	Managers use the budget to guide operations in order to derive profits.

- fixed costs—costs that do not change due to volume
- variable costs—costs that vary in relation to volume
- semivariable costs—costs that vary with volume but not directly
- step costs—costs that vary with specific volume levels

The point of flexible budgeting is to incorporate these cost concepts in the budget. For example, a nursing unit may discover that its variable costs rise significantly with volume:

Fexible Budget for Nursing Program

Number of Patients Served:	1,000	2,000	3,000
Fixed Costs	$24,000	$24,000	$24,000
Variable Costs	3,500	7,000	10,500
Semivariable Costs	1,000	1,200	1,400
TOTAL	$28,500	$32,200	$35,900

The fixed costs for the salaries of two licensed vocational nurses remains the same regardless of volume. The variable costs (e.g., for supplies) are directly proportional to volume. As the number of patients served changes from 1,000 to 2,000, the variable costs also double. The semivariable costs rise by $200 for every increment of 1,000 patients served.

The point of flexible budgeting is to explicitly incorporate cost behavior in budgeting. Hence a static budget of $32,200 fails to cover the expenses of the situation where 3,000 patients are served. The nursing program experiences a shortfall of $3,700 ($35,900 − $32,200 = $3,700). The organization is reaping added revenues because it has served 1,000 more patients. However, this fact may be little consolation to the nursing program unless it is allocated additional funds to cover the variable and semivariable costs.

Another means for understanding variable budgeting is to consider changes that take place in volume, price, and quantity.[25,26] For example, any nursing unit, program, or department may discover that it has exceeded its budget because of variations in volume, price, or quantity:

Variance in Expenditures on Nursing Services = Volume Variance + Price Variance + Quantity Variance

Unless these variances are accounted for each month or during fiscal periods, the nursing program's or department's budget cannot match reality. In cases where the variances are favorable, the net result is overfunding. However, when an excessive number of patient days are served, prices (i.e., salaries) rise, or an increase in the amount of nursing hours per patient day results; the net effect is a mismatch between budgeted and actual performance. These variances for volume and price are depicted in Figures 5–3 and 5–4. The quantity variance is calculated as the difference between the flexible budget for nursing salaries (i.e., Figure 5–3) and the subflexible budget for nursing salaries (i.e., Figure 5–4).

The problem confronting nursing administrators is to rectify the variances (if feasible) as soon as possible. Each month (year) results in a mismatch between

Volume Variance = Difference between Expected and Actual Production of Services by a
Nursing Unit, Program, or Department

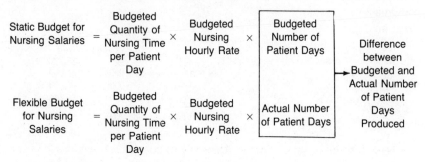

Figure 5–3 Illustration of Volume Variance

Source: Health Care Management Review, Vol. 10, No. 4, pp. 21–34, Aspen Publishers, Inc., © Fall
1985.

Price Variance = Difference between Expected and Actual Price of an Input to the
Production of Services by a Nursing Unit, Program, or Department

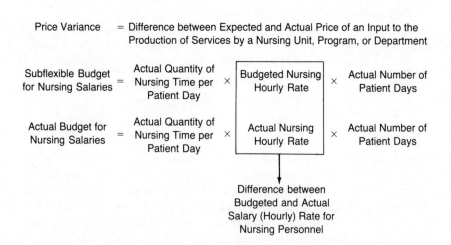

Figure 5–4 Illustration of Price Variance

Source: Health Care Management Review, Vol. 10, No. 4, pp. 21–34, Aspen Publishers, Inc., © Fall
1985.

budgeted and actual levels. Either budgets are altered to reflect the changes or year-end performance will be decidedly off target. Flexible budgeting, therefore, is a proactive approach to managing. It requires that nursing administrators and other managers with budget authority identify variances and then implement strategies that minimize the negative consequences of the variances. By accounting for budget variances on a monthly basis, the organization is better able to allocate resources in achieving its goals.

To illustrate the power of flexible budgeting, consider the following performance statistics encountered in the nursing department at Retreat Hospital:

	Budgeted	*Actual*
Number of Patient Days	6,000	7,380
Cost of Nursing Services per Hour	$15.00	$13.50
Nursing Hours per Patient Day	5.09	6.00

The number of patient days increased from a projected figure of 6,000 to 7,380 due to a successful promotional campaign undertaken by Retreat's marketing department. Meanwhile, the cost of nursing care per hour fell due to turnover among senior staff (who had expensive salaries), hiring of new graduates as replacements, and the rising supply of nurses in Retreat's community (which has lowered the salary structure). Concomitantly, the number of nursing hours delivered per patient day has risen because of the inexperience of the new hires.

The question is whether Retreat has exceeded its budgeted allocation for nursing services. Part of the rationale for budget variances is described above, but can Retreat be flexible enough to adjust its operations for the deviations from the budget projections? The answer to these questions is ascertained by examining the variances themselves.

From Figure 5–3 the volume variance is calculated as follows:

Budgeted Nursing Time		Budgeted Hourly Rate		Budgeted Patient Days		
5.09	×	$15.00	×	6,000	=	$458,100
					Volume Variance	
Budgeted Nursing Time		Budgeted Hourly Rate		Actual Patient Days		
5.09	×	$15.00	×	7,380	=	$563,643

This volume variance is viewed as *unfavorable* because it results in more nursing costs than budgeted (i.e., $563,463 − $458,100 = $105,363). Obviously, assessment of volume variances depends on perspective. From a total organizational perspective this variance is favorable; but from a budget perspective it results in an unanticipated deviation.

Using Figure 5–4, the price variance is calculated as:

Actual Nursing Time		Budgeted Hourly Rate		Actual Patient Days		
6.00	×	$15.00	×	7,380	=	$664,200
						Price Variance
Actual Nursing Time		Actual Hourly Rate		Actual Patient Days		
6.00	×	$13.50	×	7,380	=	$597,780

This price variance is viewed as *favorable* because the actual total cost of nursing care is lower than budgeted. This was primarily the result of the lower salary rate paid to nurses. In this case, the nursing department has some flexibility ($664,200 − $597,780 = $66,420) in meeting its budget objectives.

The quantity variance measures the difference in actual nursing time (in hours per patient day) versus budgeted nursing hours. This difference must be associated with actual volume and budgeted hourly rate:

Actual Nursing Time		Budgeted Hourly Rate		Actual Patient Days		
6.00	×	$15.00	×	7,380	=	$664,200
						Quantity Variance
Budgeted Nursing Time		Budgeted Hourly Rate		Actual Patient Days		
5.09	×	$15.00	×	7,380	=	$563,463

The nursing department has an *unfavorable* quantity (of nursing hours) variance of $664,200 − $563,463 = $100,737. It results from the inefficiency of the new nurses who spent more actual time per patient in delivering care (i.e., 6.00 hours) than was originally budgeted (i.e., 5.09 hours).

The overall profile emerging on performance in the nursing department is determined by the following results:

Volume Variance	=	$105,363	Unfavorable (−)
Price Variance	=	66,420	Favorable (+)
Quantity Variance	=	100,737	Unfavorable (−)
Nursing Department Variance	=	$139,680	Unfavorable (−)

Combining the variances, it is clear that the nursing department has exceeded its budget by $139,680. In part, this budget was violated due to more patient days (i.e., 7,380) over which the department had little or no control. Direct gains of $66,420 were made due to the lower salary of new staff nurses, but this could not compensate for their inefficiency.

At this point, the director of nursing must formulate a logical plan for improving the productivity of the nursing staff in order to reduce the quantity variance. Attention to this factor should help to improve actual performance and better address budgeted targets. Management control is possible because flexible budgeting has pinpointed the consequences of inefficient service delivery in specific dollar terms.

DECENTRALIZING NURSING BUDGETS

Nursing administrators are increasingly becoming involved in plans for decentralized budgets, not only within health care organizations but also within their departments.[27,28] The intent of these plans is to incorporate nursing staff in the planning and budgeting process. Ostensibly this should lead to greater control because those staff responsible for formulating the budget are more cognizant of its determination, including the trade-offs that must be made to attain targeted performance levels. There are many variations on how decentralized budgeting can occur. However, a useful approach is for the director of nursing to delegate budgeting responsibility to the head nurses and assistant head nurses.[29] Once this occurs, the head nurses may seek input from staff nurses. The overall result can be the staff's greater commitment to budgets.

These proposals for incorporating staff nurses in the budgeting process are particularly crucial in view of the high nursing costs in most health care organizations. Although inclusion of the nursing staff does require time (and hence produces more costs), the advantage of commitment to mutually determined performance objectives offers a substantial rationale for decentralized budgeting. As usual, decentralized budgeting is not a panacea. A nursing administrator must carefully assess the skills, experience, and personality of nurses who would be incorporated in the budgeting process before deciding to decentralize.

NOTES

1. J. Keith Deisenioth, "Understanding the Budget Process," *Topics in Health Care Financing* 5 (Summer 1979): 1–17.
2. Russell C. Swansburg, "The Nursing Budget," *Supervisor Nurse* 9 (June 1978): 40–47.
3. Thomas A. Gavin, "Financial Accounting and Internal Control Functions Pursued by Hospital Boards," *Healthcare Financial Management* 38 (September 1984): 26–32.
4. John D. Stairs and John R. Coleman, "Survey Shows Budgeting Art Improved in Hospitals," *Hospital Financial Management* 33 (October 1979): 52–54, 56–58, 60–61.

5. Michael Kingsbury, "Budget Model Applications," *Topics in Health Care Financing* 5 (Summer 1979): 95–105.

6. Thomas P. Herzog, "Productivity: Fighting the Battle of the Budget," *Nursing Management* 16 (January 1985): 30–34.

7. Robert C. Nauert, "An Effective Way to Plan and Budget for Available Resources," *Healthcare Financial Management* 38 (September 1984): 64–68.

8. Constance Lloyd and Judy Ford, "Developing a Budget: A Vital Tool for Success," *Group Practice Journal* 29 (December 1980): 7–9.

9. "More Hospitals Budget, and More Complexly," *Hospitals* 53 (October 16, 1979): 28, 30, 34.

10. Jane Farrar Granshaw, "The Computer-assisted Budget," *Topics in Health Care Financing* 10 (Fall 1983): 9–26.

11. "Departmental Input Helps Stabilize Budgets," *Hospitals* 56 (February 1, 1982): 39, 48–49.

12. Frances M. Hoffman, "Projecting Supply Expenses," *Journal of Nursing Administration* 15 (June 1985): 21–24.

13. Charles E. Housley, "Budgeting at the Supervisor's Level," *Hospital Topics* 54 (March/April 1976): 6, 8, 11.

14. Walton M. Hancock and Paul A. Fuhs, "The Relationship Between Nurse Staffing Policies and Nursing Benefits," *Health Care Management Review* 9 (Fall 1984): 21–26.

15. Woodford W. King, "Budgeting for Contractual Allowances," *Hospital Financial Management* 35 (January 1981): 58–59.

16. Charles H. Byington, "Gross A/R: No Management Measure," *Hospital Financial Management* 33 (June 1979): 32, 34, 36.

17. James E. Bolinger, "Payment Patterns," *Hospital Financial Management* 34 (March 1980): 70.

18. Edward Zak, "Implementing and Maintaining Flexible Budgeting," *Topics in Health Care Financing* 5 (Summer 1979): 85–94.

19. William H. Holder, "Hospital Budgeting: State of the Art," *Hospital and Health Services Administration* 23 (Spring 1978): 51–59.

20. Donald H. Sweeney, "Flexible Budgeting: The Great Escape," *Hospital Financial Management* 29 (August 1975): 36–38.

21. Terrence J. Scott, "Variable Budgeting: To Accurately Monitor a Hospital's Performance," *Hospital Financial Management* 34 (May 1980): 42–48.

22. Robert D. Rogers, "Preparation of the Budget and the Flexible Operating Plan," *Topics in Health Care Financing* 5 (Summer 1979): 19–32.

23. Ronald Layman, "Flexible Budgeting for Small Hospitals," *Hospital Financial Management* 34 (October 1980): 64–65.

24. William W. Holder and Jan Williams, "Better Cost Control with Flexible Budgeting and Variance Analysis," *Hospital Financial Management* 30 (January 1976) 12–20.

25. Steven A. Finkler, "Flexible Budget Variance Analysis Extended to Patient Acuity and DRGs," *Health Care Management Review* 10 (Fall 1985): 21–34.

26. Edward J. Sorenson, "Flexible Budgeting—Easier Than You Think," *Hospital Financial Management* 33 (April 1979): 40–43.

27. Joan Nietz Althaus, Nancy McDonald Hardyck, Patricia Blair Pierce, and Marilyn S. Rodgers, "Decentralized Budgeting: Holding the Purse Strings, Part I," *Journal of Nursing Administration* 12 (May 1982): 15–20.

28. Jane A. Fanning and Ruth Busch Lovett, "Decentralization Reduces Nursing Administration Budget," *Journal of Nursing Administration* 15 (May 1985): 19–24.

29. Joan Nietz Althaus, Nancy McDonald Hardyck, Patricia Blair Pierce, and Marilyn S. Rodgers, "Decentralized Budgeting: Holding the Purse Strings, Part II," *Journal of Nursing Administration* 12 (June 1982): 34–38.

Chapter 6

Working Capital Management

At the very heart of the financial operations of any health care organization is the day-to-day management of assets and liabilities. Without careful attention to these operations, an organization would never be able to reach its long-run objectives successfully. And yet, like other management functions, financing theory and practice often neglect current operations. This problem has been exacerbated in the health care field by third party payment policies that effectively removed the threat of immediate financial insolvency.[1] However, even with prospective payment the problem of achieving financial goals is still seen as a long-run problem of matching services with demand and revenue. Thus, day-to-day control of operations is often downplayed.

Nursing administrators are usually very sensitive to issues of current operations. They are generally responsible for establishing staffing schedules, monitoring consumption of supplies related to the provision of services, maintaining a core staff without relying excessively on expensive nursing pools or overtime, obtaining support from ancillary staff that can be used in the most efficient manner, and directing program staff toward effective and efficient attainment of work unit, program, or department goals. Although these activities appear to be nonfinancial in nature, the contrary is true. It is the rigorous use of current assets that reflects a financial orientation.

In order for nursing administrators to acquire knowledge of working capital management concepts, it is essential that they broaden their vision of the tasks they routinely complete. They need to see the financial management function as part of their role as nursing administrators. In many respects, they have been undertaking these responsibilities as a normal part of their job. There is probably no other problem as significant as failing to envision the nursing management function as compatible with financial management.

Nurse administrators have a variety of strengths that can contribute to the financial operations of a health care organization. More so than financial staff members, the nurse administrator usually has extensive *line* experience. Nursing leaders have spent substantial time, usually years, involved in clinical care responsibilities. They have been responsible for directing, leading, motivating, and evaluating staff nurses and ancillary personnel. More likely than not, they have also been extensively involved with department heads, program directors, and management representatives. The give and take of this experience is invaluable because the nurse administrator knows what will work and what will fail in management interventions. But, to make this knowledge truly useful to the health care organization, it must be integrated within a logical framework for managing functional operations. This is where a financial management perspective is needed.

Although the financial staff holds superior technical knowledge of managing current operations, it is still essential to translate those concepts into practice. Here is where the nurse administrator can make an invaluable contribution.

THE NATURE OF WORKING CAPITAL IN HEALTH CARE FACILITIES

In most business organizations the term working capital has been used to indicate current assets. As raw materials and resources (such as labor) are brought together they produce certain goods and services. The net result is the creation of current assets. Current assets that are not sold will accumulate (e.g., inventory). Balanced against the growth of the assets is the accumulation of debts or liabilities resulting from the conversion of raw materials into a final product. Thus working capital is reduced as current liabilities are paid.

The working capital concept is often used interchangeably with the term current assets. Yet, the financial account must be balanced. Liabilities incurred in generating assets offset those assets. Hence, a judicious reading of the production of goods and services indicates that current assets are only *one* aspect of working capital. For this reason some financial managers will use the term net working capital to differentiate between current assets and current liabilities. Net working capital would include all current assets less all current liabilities.

The terminology is critical because of overlap and room for misinterpretation. Working capital management is the management of all current assets (e.g., cash, marketable securities, receivables, inventories, and so forth) and all current liabilities (e.g., accounts payable, notes payable, provision for federal income tax, and so forth). Because the acquisition of capital to undertake current operations often requires long-term financing, it is necessary to include long-run financing decisions within the purview of working capital management. Here is where current operations relate to overall financial management. Working capital management is not just an insulated concept but an integral part of a total financial plan. Long-run sources of capital are usually needed to fund current operations. Thus, working capital management does not focus exclusively on current operations but must acknowledge broader financial concerns as well.

Consistent with the American Hospital Association, the Health Care Financial Management Association, and other health care associations interested in financial operation, working capital can be further defined as:[2]

Working Capital = Current Assets − Current Liabilities
Working Capital Requirements =

- Funds to cover expenses during the time between when services are provided and when charges are collected
- Funds to build or maintain inventories
- Funds to provide for rising premiums on prepaid insurance
- Funds to provide cash or other liquid assets for unanticipated needs

This delineation is useful for three reasons. First, it reinforces the definition of working capital as consisting of both current assets and current liabilities. Second, it specifies the required funds needed to maintain current operations. Third, it introduces the concepts of charges and third party payment that make the management of working capital in health care organizations unique compared with other businesses.

INTEGRATING THIRD PARTY PAYMENT

Inevitably there is a lag between when services are delivered and when charges are collected. The main exception to this rule is the cash-paying customer who represents a small percentage of all patients. Therefore health care organizations must not only anticipate a significant lag between when they deliver services and when they are paid, but also between when services are delivered and when a bill can actually be prepared. Once the internal billing process is established, the health care organization still confronts the processing time required by the third party payer. It is apparent that the management of working capital must rely extensively on managing cash flows and preparing cash supplements (e.g., short-term financing or cash reserves) to account for a high degree of uncertainty and general delay within the system.

Since charges not yet paid are accounted for as receivables, it is important to monitor the aging of these receivables. This allows not only a check on the extent to which bills are being paid, but also helps in planning for short-term financing of the temporary deficit. The typical accounts receivable aging analysis could be formulated around the following format:

Age of Account in Days

Account	0–30	31–60	61–90	91–120	121–150	151–180	over 180	TOTAL
Medicare	____	____	____	____	____	____	____	____
Medicaid	____	____	____	____	____	____	____	____
Blue Cross	____	____	____	____	____	____	____	____
Commercial	____	____	____	____	____	____	____	____
Self-pay	____	____	____	____	____	____	____	____
Other	____	____	____	____	____	____	____	____

Although each health care organization will have its own set of circumstances, it is useful to remember that by grouping the accounts it is possible to ascertain which accounts are habitually late in fulfilling their obligations. These accounts should receive added managerial attention because ultimately they are the impetus behind short-term financial planning and fund acquisition. It may be possible to negotiate directly with late accounts and thereby circumvent the acquisition of short-term loans to cover expenses in a given period.

BLENDING CURRENT AND LONG-RUN OPERATIONS

If working capital is managed correctly, decisions must be made about how to blend current operations with long-run operations. The policies that are selected must not sacrifice either current or long-run operations. Therefore, blending current and long-run operations essentially means that decisions on the management of current assets must be attuned to anticipated revenues and anticipated drawdowns on those revenues. Any shortfall implies an additional analysis of policies on return on investment and charitable contributions as well as other vital organizational goals.

These ideas are very important as a result of the diversity of revenue sources within health care organizations. For example, a hospital must plan its working capital requirements around its patient care services. It receives revenue for providing these services from many sources that ultimately influence cash flow and hence working capital management. However, revenue from providing patient care is not the only source of revenue to most hospitals. It is the additional sources of funds that help health care managers blend current and long-run operations.

An organization must also resist consistently using debt to fund its current operations; otherwise it will threaten its long-run survival. Therefore, it is best to use revenues from current operations to fund current operations, and to use long-run financing (and incremental surpluses from operations) to fund long-run capital projects. The question that remains is what revenues to use in maintaining this balance of short- and long-run operations.

Nurse administrators may have been exposed to many of the nonpatient care sources of revenue that can be utilized to reduce the problems in managing cash flows. These sources include other operating revenue and nonoperating revenue:

Illustrations of Other Operating Revenue (i.e., Nonpatient Care Revenue)

- Rental of space
- Cafeteria sales to staff, guests, medical staff, visitors
- Charges for telephone or television use (or other activities) by staff, visitors, patients
- Recycling receipts from metal scrap, radiology supplies, food wastes, or other salvage
- Sales from gift shops, parking lots, vending machines, or other service programs
- Special services to staff (e.g., pharmaceutical supplies to employees)
- Research grants, gifts, or subsidies
- Educational tuition or fees
- Membership fees (e.g., for a health promotion program)
- Charges for nonpatient packages of care (e.g., seminar on natural births)

Illustrations of Nonoperating Revenue

- Gifts, grants, or donations for which there is no special use defined (i.e., an unrestricted donation)
- Interest on unrestricted endowments
- Volunteer services
- Gain on property or equipment sold

The purpose in listing these sources of other operating revenue and nonoperating revenue is to demonstrate that there is a wide variety of additional sources of revenue. The imaginative use of revenues helps balance short-term operations with long-run goals.

Balancing current operations with long-run operations also means reaching a decision on the required rate of return on equity invested. Essentially this means that a surplus (i.e., net income) that reaches a predetermined rate must be made from current operations. When expenses exceed revenues, the return on the invested capital decreases. However, even with an operating surplus, the level of the surplus may be lower than is preferred. Hence a health care organization must consciously plan for what the surplus should be and then strive to keep current operations in line with this preestablished goal.

Many third party payers are experiencing difficulty in ascertaining a correct operating surplus for hospitals. Medicare's DRG payment system has undergone several years of analysis and discussion in exploring allowable rates for capital investment. By returning to industries such as the steel and automotive manufacturers it is possible to understand what happens when capital is not reinvested in plant and equipment. Eventually these organizations cannot compete in terms of price or product because their plant and equipment is too outdated to respond to the demands of the marketplace. Hospitals have experienced a similar impact due to failure to reinvest in capital assets (e.g., facility). They were unprepared when prospective pricing clamped down on capital reimbursement.

Return on current operations is ultimately an issue of greatest significance to *every* health care organization, whether it is public, nonprofit, or investor-owned. The current operating surplus is effectively the return on investment. The special term used to denote the surplus from current operations is the operating margin:

Operating Margin = Total Operating Revenue −
Current Operating Requirements
Where:
Total Operating Revenue = (Patient Care Revenue + Other
Operating Revenue) − Deductions
Current Operating Requirements = Operating expenses for patient service, teaching,
and research

The operating margin can be depicted in the following manner:

Working Capital Funds Required		
Cash	$ 10,000	
Accounts Receivable	140,000	
Payment of Long-Term Debt	200,000	
Accounts Payable	(70,000)	
Net Working Capital Funds		$280,000
Capital Funds Required		
Renovation of Ward C	$200,000	
New Equipment	75,000	
Restricted Funds for Plant Replacement	(50,000)	
Net Capital Funds		225,000
Funds Required		$505,000
Depreciation		$400,000
OPERATING MARGIN		105,000
Sources of Funds		$ 505,000

Working capital requirements incorporate an operating margin that provides a return on investment after accounting for all taxes. The operating margin essentially covers all of the working capital funds (in the example above: cash, accounts receivable, payment of long-term debt, and accounts payable), capital funds (in the example above: renovation, new equipment, and restricted funds), and where appropriate, a dividend to investors.

MANAGING CURRENT ASSETS

Half of the working capital equation involves the management of current assets. Like any organization, a health care organization is concerned with maximizing its control over current assets—especially cash. The sooner accounts receivable are collected, the sooner the health care organization can reinvest those funds. The task of managing current assets is more complex for health care organizations than other organizations due to third party payers. Since third parties interface with thousands of health care providers, they tend to set the operating rules and policies. The individual provider has little power to enforce its desires short of professional lobbying (e.g., through professional associations) or through legal means. Ultimately few gains are made.

For this reason, the management of current assets usually reverts to that which the health care organization can control best—its internal operations. It can establish policies for managing cash.[3] It can be judicious in investing cash reserves in marketable securities. Above all, it must formulate a plan for managing accounts receivable including billing practices, collections, and timely investment of those collections.[4] Inventory and supplies must be carefully planned to avoid unnecessary consumption, pilferage, or decay. Additionally, the organization must assess its position on periodic receipt of charges from third parties versus true billing.[5]

For the nurse administrator there are innumerable opportunities to participate in these activities. In some cases the nurse administrator will serve only as a representative for nursing services because the nursing department can contribute minimally toward resolving a current assets problem. For example, the nursing administrator may participate in a financial staff meeting on how to improve collections and provide thoughts on how nursing can help the organization profile the reluctant payer. In other cases the nurse administrator will take a leading role. For example, the nursing director may convey to other department heads the unique inventory control practices nursing has implemented to hold down missing medications or other supplies.

CASH MANAGEMENT

Cash is the most liquid of all assets and therefore must receive special attention not only to maximize its values but to protect against its loss.[6] Cash can be found in many forms other than just currency. Checks, temporary or demand deposits, and similar liquid instruments constitute cash, while specified term deposits or other short-term securities constitute investments. Nurse administrators who closely examine this definition of cash will realize that they and their staff may seldom have opportunities to be involved in cash management. An exception may be the nurse who is given added responsibilities beyond the clinical area for helping in administration or a business office. For example, nurses in medical clinics are sometimes requested to transport liquid or negotiable assets such as cash and checks to banks for deposit. This may be a regular responsibility they fulfill because they are viewed as trustworthy.

The failure to establish an effective control system at all points at which cash is handled is probably the single most important reason why health care organizations experience cash losses. There must be checks and double checks on the entire system. But cash management just does not end with control. There is a critical planning component as well.[7] Cash must be treated as a security with time value— it can depreciate in value unless it is invested in a manner that will provide interest on the principle.

Nurse administrators should also be familiar with cash management in order to participate effectively in the financial operations of the organization as they acquire greater managerial responsibilities. They may be able to bring a new perspective in how to avoid misappropriations, or they may be able to add insight into how to improve timely cash inflows. It is also essential that they prepare themselves for the time when they are delegated responsibility for managing cash inflows and outflows.

Cash is an asset that consumes a disproportionate amount of time for its total dollar amount relative to other assets. Yet like so many management variables, it is possible to establish a general policy for cash receipts, temporary investment, and eventual disbursement without any undue results. The point is that the effective manager strives to gain optimum performance from all assets. Cash should be treated as any other asset—and more. Therefore, it is ultimately the responsibility of health care managers to exercise extensive caution in cash management. Cash receipts and disbursements are the lifeblood of an organization's operations and should be treated with appropriate caution and respect.

An effective cash management program seeks to accomplish several objectives:[8,9]

- Control must establish standards and a basis for evaluation under which the productivity (return) of the asset can be ascertained. Cash must be effectively used 100 percent of the time.
- Plans for fulfilling short-run and long-run organizational cash needs must be established and implemented.

- Plans for secure handling of cash receipts for deposit should be created and put into operation.
- Control must ensure that there are adequate safeguards to prevent misappropriation and incorrect disbursement.
- Plans for contingency needs should be developed to explain where, when, and how supplemental funds will be obtained. Standards must be established beforehand to determine what constitutes a legitimate crisis worthy of emergency efforts.

The starting point for any cash management program is to determine management's commitment to a maximum return on the asset. If this commitment is made, it will be necessary to maintain minimum balances in low-interest demand deposits (i.e., savings accounts) and checking accounts. Temporary surplus cash must be immediately invested in short-term investments (e.g., certificate of deposits, treasury bills, money market accounts). Borrowing will be avoided whenever possible because the organization will experience added expenses (i.e., interest) for the use of someone else's money. All cash discounts will be taken advantage of when they offer a favorable return to the organization.[10]

Planning Cash Needs

Cash needs are the prime worry of many chief financial officers. They know that if they fine-tune operations excessively it is feasible that cash on hand will not meet demands. This is generally bothersome only because it implies that the health care organization cannot pay its bills. However, in most cases there are adequate reserves in short-term investments to resolve the problem immediately. What is most distasteful is the *implication* that financial health is less than perfect, and that the plan for fulfilling cash needs was imperfect. These occasional occurrences will undoubtedly afflict every financial officer at one point or another.

Nurse administrators may wonder exactly how these plans are made in the first place to allow low balances in cash accounts. How can operations be run at the razor's edge with respect to amount of cash on hand and still maintain short-run solvency? The answer is the cash plan and its forecast.

A typical method for estimating cash flows is to assess annual cash receipts and disbursements to ascertain trends. This method can be used with several years' data. The strength of this model is the reliance on actual past results. Its weakness is an inability to account for recent changes (e.g., bed expansion) or for anticipated changes (e.g., in third party payment). The model may analyze the following data over several years in projecting estimated receipts and disbursements for a coming fiscal year.

	January	February	···	December	Total Average
Cash on Hand	$ 80,714	$ 77,142	···	$ 65,237	$ 76,456
Cash Receipts					
Patient Care	417,329	400,201	···	394,700	409,131
Nonpatient Care	86,543	92,741	···	80,003	84,882
Total Cash Receipts	503,872	492,942	···	474,703	494,013
Total Cash Available	584,586	570,084	···	539,940	570,469
Cash Payments					
Accounts Payable	334,215	300,003	···	298,762	311,007
Payroll	104,200	114,895	···	122,676	113,999
Taxes	8,798	10,213	···	11,117	10,798
Funded Debt	10,000	10,000	···	10,000	10,000
Total Cash Payments	457,213	435,111	···	442,555	445,804
Net	$127,373	$134,973	···	$ 97,385	124,665

In the example it is easy to see that cash on hand averaged $76,456. This is a substantial amount that is only being supported by the net cash proceeds from operations. In this situation there is a favorable problem; that is, the health care manager must invest excess cash due to the high amount of cash generated by operations. It is far better to be in this position than facing deficits and borrowing to float operations until net cash proceeds can be obtained.

Much of this planning and record keeping can be completed on personal or microcomputers. Many financial management software packages available today make this financial forecasting easier than in the past. However, this does not relieve nurse administrators from knowing the basics around which those packages are formulated, nor does it relieve them of the responsibility to adjust the package to fit their specific situation.

Nurse administrators should recognize the value of the programs to predict alternative financial scenarios. The packages typically allow users to change variable values by asking "what if" questions. With these capabilities the nurse administrator or any other user need only carefully contemplate how variables will change and by what magnitude. Then these new assumptions are entered into the programs to attain a fresh perspective on future operations. However, this sort of alternative scenario-building can rapidly get out of control, since the possibilities are infinite.

Another useful cash plan relates to long-run planning for capital projects and payment of debt. This financial planning is directly linked to capital budgeting. However, it deserves special emphasis here because of a prevalent failure of health care organizations in the past.

Many health care facilities, particularly hospitals, were guilty of not replenishing their capital assets through funding from current operations. Without an emphasis on cost control (due to cost-pass-through reimbursement), hospitals simply set little or nothing aside for expansion or replacement. Whenever these capital requirements became immediate, a hospital merely raised its rates, sought philanthropy, or obtained a government grant. With those times past, health care organizations now have to fund from current operations. Consequently they will increasingly need to project cash requirements over several years:

	Year 1	Year 2	Year 3	Year 4	Year 5
Cash Expenditures:					
Major Equipment					
Purchases	$115,000	$ 95,000	$ 95,000	$ 95,000	$ 95,000
Addition to					
Building #1	323,000				
Lease Payment on					
Lithotripter	45,000	45,000	45,000	45,000	
Surgicenter					
Construction	110,000	110,000			
Parking Lot					
Procedure	10,000	10,000	70,000		
Total	603,000	260,000	210,000	140,000	95,000
Additions to					
Working Capital	40,000	37,000	39,000	38,000	40,000
Debt Payments					
Revenue Bonds	78,000	79,000	81,000	83,000	85,000
New Financing			30,000	32,000	33,000
Total Cash					
Required	$721,000	$376,000	$360,000	$293,000	$253,000

This projected cash plan must be reconciled with the anticipated revenue inflows. Presumably there will be added revenue streams attached to the construction associated with Building #1, the lithotripter, and the surgicenter. Those sources should have already been integrated with the cash flow plans of the organization. The critical aspect of projecting cash requirements is to create a basis from which financing of short-run cash needs can be predicted and fulfilled. It has value in establishing a schedule for financing *some* long-term obligations; but the capital budget is usually responsible for capital expenditures. Finally, notice that cash is used in planning for both short-run and long-run obligations.

Planning Secure Cash Handling

Secure cash handling depends on planning around four main factors:

1. Banks and other investment institutions that maintain cash accounts
2. The accounting department that records the cash transaction and maintains the resources for periodic audits

3. The business office that receives the transaction and over which the chief cashier should exercise the first line of control
4. Top management and financial staff who have decision-making authority to influence where cash is deposited in order for it to earn interest

The key is to remove as many people from handling cash as possible and to introduce dual reporting to the greatest extent possible. This is why most organizations rely on a centralized office for receipts. It reduces the opportunities for misappropriation. Most organizations also try to introduce reconciliation of funds as a responsibility separate from handling of cash itself. Bringing these techniques together with random audits should be sufficient to protect most cash flows, although managers should never become complacent about their systems—it is the tendency to be satisfied with current operations that invites abuse.

Many good ideas have been suggested for managing cash receipts and disbursements from the standpoint of security. Following are a few illustrations of the techniques for controlling losses of cash:

Receipts	*Disbursements*
• Cash received should be recorded, and periodically these records should be reconciled with deposit slips.	• All disbursements except petty cash should be made by check.
• Cash receipts should be deposited daily in a single amount.	• All petty cash disbursements should require dual signatures.
• Employees handling cash should be periodically relieved by an individual capable of auditing the function.	• All checks should require dual signatures.
• All personnel should be bonded.	• Checks should be numbered and a sequence maintained.
• Bank deposits should be reconciled with cash receipt slips.	• Those managing cash disbursements should not be handling cash receipts.
	• After a check is voided or payment is made, the check should be retained and properly filed.

These lists are not meant to be exhaustive, but merely illustrative of the detail that is required to properly complete the secure management of cash. Through techniques such as these—and many other control procedures—it is possible to protect the organization's most liquid asset.

Planning Effective Return on Funds

At its greatest extension, cash management requires in-depth planning to achieve an effective return on funds. It has been suggested, for example, that by formulating a daily cash report it is possible to minimize the funds tied up in checks written but not yet cashed.[11] This "float" represents a legitimate source of funds for investment that should not be forgone. Other authorities have viewed this as a trade-off between short costs and long costs.[12] Short costs represent the cost of obtaining short-run financing to cover a shortage in cash. Long costs are the returns that could have been earned had the excess cash been invested in the first place. Clearly the key is to synchronize cash receipts and disbursements to maximize the return on all cash funds.

THE ROLE OF MARKETABLE SECURITIES

Assuming that a health care organization has carefully planned its cash arrangement to the point that it has reduced its float and it is prepared to invest its funds to maximum advantage, what alternatives does it have to choose from? There are many, including:

- U.S. Treasury bills, certificates, notes (T-bills)
- Prime commercial paper (a written agreement to repay a sum of money at a given interest rate)
- Negotiable certificates of deposit that have varying maturity dates
- Governmental notes
- Demand deposits (savings accounts)
- Corporate stocks
- Corporate notes and bonds
- Certificates of deposit (CDs)

Other short-term investment opportunities continue to present themselves as lenders seek ingenious ways to attract borrowers.

The decision to select a short-run marketable security hinges on risk and yield. Since health care organizations are usually not in a position of making a substantial return on excess cash, it is best to assume a conservative posture in which a low return is accepted. Only when funds will be available for an extended period of time is it appropriate to consider pursuing a higher return that increases the risk of not having ready access to cash. The last thing that a financial manager wants is to have to borrow funds to cover cash shortages. The rate of the borrowed funds will be higher than the return on the investment that has not reached maturity.

In reaching a policy on marketable securities and cash management, it is often suggested that weekly net cash flows be estimated.[13] A variation on the monthly report for cash requirements can be used in this estimate:

Account	Week Ended XX/XX/XX	Month-to-Date Actual	Predicted
Cash Balance	$ 8,970	$ 36,888	$ 35,500
Cash Receipts			
Patient Care	16,140	48,754	45,000
Nonpatient Care	7,760	17,321	17,000
Total	23,900	66,075	62,000
Cash Payments			
Accounts Payable	9,933	10,212	10,000
Payroll	10,115	30,422	30,000
Inventory	675	2,210	1,500
Capital Expenditures	1,211	3,698	1,500
Total	21,934	46,542	43,000
Ending Cash Balance	$ 1,966	$ 19,533	$ 19,000

As usual, any monthly report is only as meaningful as the use it receives.[14] The point in creating the reports is to assess the progress in cash balances in order to invest them at the earliest possible time at the highest possible yield.

ACCOUNTS RECEIVABLE

Until all charges are paid in full, a health care organization has merely a cluster of accounts receivable that represent frozen assets. Like any business, health care organizations must seek timely payment of these charges so that they in turn can pay their own bills. As experience generally dictates, the longer these bills remain uncollected, the longer it will take to collect them. Bad debts (an operating expense) rise with an increasing length of time since first billing.[15] Consequently nurse managers should recognize that exceptional attention should be directed toward controlling accounts receivable.

Fortunately health care organizations have considerable help in their attempts at getting bills paid. Third party payment offers a tremendous advantage in providing secure reimbursement for services delivered. Thus, an organization is less concerned than other businesses with validating the creditworthiness of its patients. However, health care organizations must document third party coverage, which does present some problems. More worrisome is the situation where an individual does not have insurance. The health care charge system is designed to maximize reimbursement cost. Without coverage for a patient, the provider faces an increasingly likely bad debt. Not only must more effort be expended in gaining payment, the probability increases that payment will never actually be made.

Another factor influencing this chain of events in accounts receivable is the attitude that health care is a right. Health care providers are expected to provide charitable care to an unspecified percentage of patients. For this reason alone, some patients either cannot pay or will not pay. This is a significant challenge in managing accounts receivable—control must be exercised to prevent receivables from becoming bad debts. Many mechanisms and safeguards can be invoked. However, the most effective starting point in managing accounts receivable occurs before a patient is admitted to the facility or before services are delivered.

Consider the normal admissions and collections processes for accounts receivable shown in Figure 6–1.[16] A patient registers and is admitted. Services are provided, followed by discharge. Once the bill is formulated, the hospital has generated accounts receivable. Since accounts receivable represent idle cash and taxable assets it is in the best interests of the health care organization to obtain collection as soon as possible. Uncollected accounts receivable represent idle dollars that are not providing a return of any magnitude. After patient discharge the hospital itself assumes the burden of managing accounts receivable. It must develop a bill that then must be sent to the patient. During this time the hospital's assets are still idle. Then the hospital must collect the bill. It is important to reiterate that as long as the account is unpaid, assets remain idle.

In contrast with the normal process for patient admission and billing, admissions-oriented accounts receivable is forward looking. It seeks to control the length of time that a health care organization's assets are tied up in the receivables stage. At the time of patient registration, the patient is counselled on the responsibilities for paying the bill incurred. At this moment the provider anticipates the eventual discharge of the patient. By anticipating a future accounts receivable at the admissions stage, the provider is able to gather information that might needlessly delay billing and collection. Foremost is the determination of coverage and pertinent addresses for billing. Documentation must be precise. Medical staff should be alerted to the policy that patients need to bring claim forms with them in order to be eligible for admission. In this manner the majority of the barriers to timely accounts receivable management can be overcome. Forms can be completed (e.g., signatures) at this time to the fullest extent possible.

Not every patient has third party coverage. In these situations it is appropriate to begin financial counselling that establishes cash deposits and time payment plans. Use of patients' commercial credit cards has grown in popularity as a method for short-term financing. In other cases it is necessary to plan monthly payments at a predetermined interest rate. Still other cases present absolutely no hope for payment and must be either written off as charitable care or routed to public assistance.

The key of admissions-oriented accounts receivable is that it anticipates discharge. Figure 6–1 indicates that after services are provided, and prior to discharge, there should be another attempt by the organization to review all

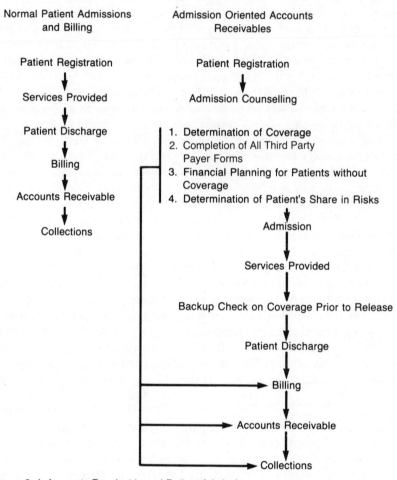

Figure 6–1 Accounts Receivable and Patient Admissions

paperwork. Have all needed signatures been obtained? Are all forms in place? Are the correct addresses available? This backup check will reinforce the admissions check. After the patient is discharged, the health care organization has little control over the completion of accounts receivable. It must use its time and power wisely to achieve good receivables management.

Billing

An account is not a receivable until it is billed. Therefore the billing department is an essential element in the process of obtaining quick coverage on accounts receivable. In order to make the billing function perform best it is necessary to implement direct control—the most effective control is achieved through a qualified, well-motivated (through pay and other rewards), and experienced staff. The director of billing must be able to devote substantial time to supervising clerks rather than allocating time solely to billing functions themselves. Furthermore, the billing supervisor must have sufficient time to assess and improve the system. Without careful reflection on where improvements can be made and how to implement them the system will remain crisis-oriented.[17]

Beyond this strategy at controlling billing, it is possible to suggest a number of recommendations that should be implemented with every billing system to ensure effective operation:[18]

- Billing should begin as soon as the patient registers. By that time the patient should already know that specific information on coverage and pertinent addresses will be gathered—there should be no surprises.

- Preestablished policies for deposits (i.e., in the event of lack of proof of adequate coverage), payment deadlines (i.e., for a time payment schedule), penalties (i.e., for failing to meet deadlines), qualifications for charitable care, and referral to other providers must be firmly adhered to in the management of billing.

- Billing supervisors should meet periodically with the chief financial officer and the chief executive officer to review the age of accounts receivable from major third party payers. The chief executive officer should contact the third party about delays in receipt of payment. Professional associations (e.g., state hospital associations) may be invoked to buttress agreements for improved operations from third party payers.

- Control logs should be used to supplement computerized processing systems. There must be a duplicate record for computerized systems in the event of system malfunction. The control log should reconcile automated entries and actual recorded services.

- Physicians should be integrated into the billing system by creating educational and inservice programs. Elicit the support of the medical director, chief executive officer, and board of directors (if necessary) to obtain cooperation from staff physicians. If necessary, the organization may terminate or suspend privileges for habitual abusers.

- A consistent, accurate reporting system on billing should be developed and used. Simply charting deficiencies does nothing about resolving those problems.

- The medical records department should clarify diagnosis on patient discharge. More third party payment is oriented toward diagnosis related payment; therefore billing must be able to ascertain principal diagnoses easily.

The preceding recommendations clearly suggest that effective billing requires attention to detail. Although nurse administrators may have few opportunities for actually managing such billing processes, there are proposed changes that would involve them extensively in patient billing.

Variable billing for hospital services that breaks down the per diem hospital charge has been proposed.[19] For example, a patient in a hospital is billed for routine services surrounding each inpatient day. There are many products that contribute to care delivered during a routine inpatient day including dietary, housekeeping, nursing services, and so forth. It is argued that nursing services are often underfunded (i.e., are allocated an insufficient budget) because they are lumped in a catchall category rather than assigned to a specific cost/profit center.[20] By identifying nursing cost centers and linking them directly to charges (i.e., revenues), it should be possible to provide more equitable funding to nursing departments. The growth of diagnosis-based reimbursement systems will provide additional reinforcement to the variable billing argument since pricing decisions should reflect the actual costs of delivering nursing care within a given diagnostic group.[21]

As the preceding discussion on patient billing shows, billing is a complex process. However, by introducing various conventions it is possible for managers to control the process and achieve better financial performance. These methods should be integrated with collections, since a bill remains unpaid unless charges are received from third parties and patients. A beginning for integrating billing and collections is to maintain a periodic report for control purposes:

	Week	Month-to-Date	Deficiencies and Suggested Action
Standard			
1. Patient Receivables by Payer:			
Blue Cross	___	_____	_____
Commercial	___	_____	_____
Medicare	___	_____	_____
Medicaid	___	_____	_____
Other	___	_____	_____
Self-pay	___	_____	_____
2. Total Receivables	___	_____	_____
3. Total Receivables Billed	___	_____	_____
4. Unbillable Patient Services	___	_____	_____
5. Total Receivables Sent to Collection	___	_____	_____

Note that this report provides weekly and monthly data on receivables as they are related to billing and collections. It presents managers with information that can be used to improve the billing and collections processes.

Collection Practices

At some point a health care provider must decide that certain accounts will not be paid unless some further action is taken. There are many strategies that can be employed to help motivate patients with unpaid accounts to begin providing a stream of revenue. Many of these strategies require external assistance, which implies that a collection may raise costs. After an account shifts from a current balance to post due status it begins to cost the organization in several ways, most notably in terms of forgone interest and possible reinvestment. For these reasons it is essential that receivables be carefully monitored for aging. The older they get the more likely that a direct intervention will have to be made.

A convenient quantitative standard has been formulated to help health care managers gauge the aging of their accounts receivable:

$$\frac{\text{Number of Days in}}{\text{Accounts Receivable}} = \frac{\text{Number of Days in the Year}}{\text{Net Patient Service Revenue} \div \text{Net Patient Receivables}}$$

The denominator consists of the accounts receivable turnover ratio. This ratio matches the proportion of receivables to revenues after deducting all discounts and allowances such as bad debts, contractual allowances, charity care, or other discounts the organization may have agreed to provide.

The actual days in accounts receivable is an artificial figure in the sense that it must relate to some standard in order to gain its value. An increasing number of days in accounts receivable suggests that accounts are remaining unpaid for a longer period of time or are not being collected. The organization is losing interest and the ability to reinvest its assets (e.g., in paying its own bills). Obviously one way of reducing the days in accounts receivable is simply to reduce the amount of receivables. This can be done by writing off unpaid accounts as bad debts. This action is fortuitous in that it improves the ratio and allows a more accurate portrayal of current accounts. However, it threatens the financial well-being of the organization if consistently followed. Revenues are not being acquired to pay for services delivered. An alternative does exist—to concentrate on improving collections.

Several components of an effective collection program can be identified:[22,23]

- It must be multifaceted. There is no single best way of managing collections because there are too many opportunities for a varied response by patients and third parties. An effective program will not rely on a single proven technique but will continue to experiment as need dictates.
- Both external collection agencies and internal staff should be used in various stages of the collection process. Internal staff should generally be involved in

the processing of documents and monitoring the age of accounts. Critical milestones should be specified and adhered to in pursuing payment. External collection agencies should usually be involved on a contractual basis to manage difficult cases. Internal resources can also be used, but there are extensive legal ramifications that must be remembered.

- Internal program staff must be trained in a legal and counselling approach to collections. Even external agencies have discovered that coercive techniques are useful in only a small number of cases. Furthermore, courts are upholding the rights of individuals when their privacy is violated by more coercive means. It appears that counselling—offering alternative financing or payment schemes, encouraging positive payment behavior rather than dwelling on payment failures—can be fruitful.
- Internal staff must be thoroughly apprised of the legal guidelines for collections. Above all there is the need to document and avoid harassment.

These ideas reflect the increasing legality of collections. Most of the actions are proscribed and require precision in order to avoid litigation. From the nurse administrator's perspective, this overview is sufficient. Recognize the sensitivity of legal issues; seek additional legal counsel if needed beyond the expertise of the director of collections.

REVENUE STREAMS

In managing current assets it is appropriate to consider how revenues are to be handled once they are received and how to request (i.e., in what form) payments from third parties in order to minimize the complexity in accounting and to place funds into productive use. These two issues represent a significant portion of managing revenue streams. It must be remembered lackadaisical practices can eventually result in substantial long-run losses on current assets and cause reactions (e.g., short-term borrowing) that may otherwise not be needed. Revenue streams can be effectively maximized through two policies—lock boxes and periodic interim payments.

Lock Boxes

With the growth of multisite health care organizations there is a question about where patients should send their payments for their accounts. A single site facility such as a hospital typically does not have a substantial problem because it serves as a central facility. But what about the group of medical clinics that serves a region, the chain of hospitals in a state, or a hospital that has several satellite clinics? Payments sent to a central site may take several days to reach the processing department. A local depository in many different geographical settings may overcome the lag in time between when payments are placed in the mail, when they are received, and when they are deposited in the bank.

A lock box is typically a post office box where arrangements have been made for deposits to be collected on a periodic basis by a bank messenger service—twice daily, daily, and so forth.[24] The bank messenger is used to minimize the time for getting payments into an interest-bearing account. At least one to two days can be reduced in processing time through such a service. Every day saved represents a gain in interest earned on receivables (now cash). With receivables running into the thousands of dollars every day, the possible interest gains are lucrative even after deducting any service charges by the bank. Once checks have been deposited, the accompanying paperwork is forwarded to the hospital where the accounts are reconciled.

Periodic Interim Payments

There are several methods by which health care providers can be paid by third party reimbursers. First is the per diem method where a set rate is determined in advance for care delivered per patient day. A variant of this method allows adjustments at a later period of time to account for higher or lower costs than the per diem—the per diem is mainly used as an estimated rate. For example, Medicare's former per diem rate for inpatient care was calculated in the following fashion:[25]

Per Diem Rate = (estimated total allowable Medicare inpatient costs +
  inpatient physician's professional component) ÷
  estimated total inpatient days

A second major rate format is the percentage of charges method, which attempts to adjust for the costs attributable to physician and hospital charges—as opposed to the number of total inpatient days. In the case of Medicare it was calculated as:

Percentage of Charges = (estimated total allowable inpatient costs +
  inpatient professional component) ÷
  estimated total inpatient charges
  for hospital and physician services

Both of these rates have the advantage of allowing providers to know in advance what their rates for services will be relative to expenditures on professional services and ability to maintain census. The primary disadvantage is the point at which payment is collected—often a considerable time after the services have been delivered. This results in a shortfall of earned interest on the liquid assets—receivables.

One means of overcoming the lag in receipt of payment for services rendered is to negotiate a periodic interim payment with a third party. Medicare is noted for promoting this concept where payment is made on a monthly or more frequent basis using an approximate reasonable cost. The cost figure is merely an estimate, but it is soundly based upon the past experience of a provider, which helps promote its accuracy. The rate and deficits (or overpayments) are then retroactively adjusted to compensate for overcharges or underpayments. It is a valuable method of helping health care providers avoid financing of accounts receivable for major third party payers. After all, the provider should not be forced to float large accounts payable of the third party—providers are not lending institutions. Providers, of course, must carefully monitor their cost versus their periodic interim rate because a final accounting does eventually occur. Overpayments must then be returned to the third party.

The advantages of periodic interim payments are readily apparent.[26] Payments are scheduled throughout the year; thus the health care provider can rely on a steady cash flow to facilitate meeting current obligations. With a consistent periodic receipt of funds the provider will be able to plan operations to a greater extent. This means that the probabilities of short-term borrowing will decrease if judicious planning is undertaken. The periodic payment helps to smooth internal operations in the sense that billing interruptions will not affect cash flow. Although billing computer hardware or software may break down in the billing department, the timely receipt of funds continues. In short, the periodic payment of estimated charges by third parties greatly enhances the management of current assets.

The advantages of periodic payment must be balanced against its disadvantages. Like all documentation for reimbursement, precision must be carefully applied to ensure that the charge report is accurate in its estimates and in the final reconciliation. The provider must ensure that it receives fair compensation for services delivered, which is best achieved by auditing billing documentation. The periodic payment also has the disadvantage of generating a single lump sum payment. This payment must then be apportioned among all accounts. Shortfalls in any coverage must be noted and reconciled retrospectively.

MANAGING CURRENT LIABILITIES

The reverse side of managing current assets is managing current liabilities. Just as there are many ideas for keeping cash productive by seeking early investment, there are corresponding ideas that are useful in minimizing the cash costs of current liabilities. These ideas go far beyond the admonition that bills should be paid as late as possible. In fact there are instances, such as patient refunds and cash discounts, when current liabilities should be paid as soon as possible once it is determined that the disbursements are legitimate.[27]

There are no set guidelines in managing current liabilities because the financial market surrounding all organizations including health care providers keeps changing. On the other hand, health care providers should recognize that their current liabilities are someone else's current assets. Therefore they will be treated in much the same manner as they treat others in current asset management.

Health care providers do have an advantage in that most of their current liabilities are personnel costs. Attention can be focused on managing personnel cost through improved staff scheduling and task analysis. With the resource-rich environment that preceded prospective payment, personnel costs in some institutions may be excessive. However, cost-effective personnel administration requires continuing attention to cutting costs whenever the organization's scope of services has changed. In the end this significant component of current liabilities is no more and no less important than other liabilities.

There are no glamorous means for cutting costs and treating current liabilities as an area for improved current asset management other than fanatical attention to detail. Nurse administrators should see current liability management as a continuous function where successive refinements improve the financial position of the health care organization but where remarkable gains are unlikely to be made unless current liabilities have been severely neglected.

SHORT-TERM DEBT

Unlike most business organizations, health care providers have four instead of three main sources for financing current obligations. These sources are invoked when current liabilities become payable and there is a shortage of cash for satisfying the obligations. With careful attention to when in the year purchases are made for supplies and equipment versus other peak demands for current liabilities (e.g., payroll) it is often possible to avoid short-term debt entirely. This is particularly true where a provider maintains a cash reserve or contingency fund to cover peak periods of cash demands. Nurse administrators should understand the relationship that exists in current liabilities and current assets. Excess current assets sit idle and do not earn the highest return possible. But their investment must be balanced against periodic demands that may arise during the year.

The three main sources of financing current obligations include:

1. Trade credit—this is a predefined period during which no interest charge is levied on purchases. Like personal charge accounts, the provider is given a specific period of time (e.g., 30 days) to pay for goods or services purchased. After the predefined time period the account accrues a service charge or interest that should be consistent with the supplier's cost of capital.

2. Short-term loans from commercial banks—this is a well-recognized form of cash that is made available in the form of a note. The provider agrees to pay the note off in a specific time period (e.g., 90 days) at a specific interest rate (e.g., ten percent). Considering the seasonal fluctuations of health care services, providers may find it convenient to employ such short-run financing. A better method is to thoroughly plan cash flow to avoid any borrowing costs.
3. Short-term securities—many corporations have used unsecured debt to finance their current operations. The short-term commercial paper is an agreement to pay back an express amount of money with an add-on for interest within a relatively short period of time (e.g., less than nine months). This commercial paper has usually been sold to commercial corporate and investment institutions.

Any or all of these three short-term financing options can be used by health care organizations to cover periodic cash shortages. Judicious financial management will usually result in reliance only on trade credits. However, a fourth alternative should be contemplated.

Accounts receivable represent a fourth form of debt power. There are basically two considerations here. First, accounts receivable represent secure collateral from which short-term loans can be gained. Accounts receivable are fairly solid collateral (depending on the age of the receivables) around which loans can be made on the potential payoff. The cash to be received represents a powerful asset because in the health care field most receivables are covered by third party payers. This is the second main consideration surrounding receivables—they are covered by solid funding sources and therefore represent relatively risk-free assets. It may be possible to negotiate interim payment agreements that can help alleviate the need for short-term debt in the first place.

PITFALLS TO AVOID IN SHORT-TERM DEBT

The biggest pitfall to avoid in using short-term debt is to substitute debt for good management practice. It is often much easier to float one or more short-term loans during the course of the year to compensate for inability or unwillingness to plan for cash flow needs during the year. The problem with this approach is that it costs the health care organization more than it should to run its current operations. By carefully scheduling disbursements before crisis situations occur, an organization can survive on its contingency reserves without further borrowing. Acquiring short-term debt is costly both in terms of transaction costs and in terms of the market interest rate. Borrowing should not be substituted for effective planning.

If nurse administrators think carefully about consistent excessive use of short-term debt they will quickly recognize another pitfall in short-term borrowing. Contemplate the health care organization that continually has to resort to short-term borrowing. After several years what has it actually done? It has used short-term debt as long-term debt. In fact, long-term debt would have provided far more favorable borrowing terms. In effect the consistent periodic supplement to current operations gradually lengthens into expensive long-term debt. It would be far better to build up contingency reserves than to continually make this sort of mistake in borrowing and managing.

A final pitfall to avoid in using short-term debt is failing to monitor the extent of restrictions imposed on the loan. There are often more restrictions on short-term debt than might otherwise be required by some lenders for other loans. The rationale for these restrictions is logical. The organization is admittedly acquiring debt in order to alleviate a significant problem. The last thing that it wants to do is create yet another problem (i.e., bankruptcy) due to these restrictions.

TRADE CREDITS

A trade credit may be available if a health care organization pays its bills on time. The terminology that accompanies trade credits is often confusing, but the following guidelines help explain this valuable source of funding for current liabilities:

- Standard Credit Terms
  - 2/10, net 30 = 2 percent discount if paid in 10 days, otherwise due in 30 days
  - 2/20, net 60 = 2 percent discount if paid in 20 days, otherwise due in 60 days
- Monthly Billing
  - EOM = Payment for all purchases made before the end of the month (usually the 25th of that month) are due in the next month
- COD = Cash on delivery
- CBD = Cash before delivery

Clearly the health care organization prefers to attain favorable terms when discounts are given and cash payments are not made for as long as possible.

Computing the effective rate of interest from trade discounts is very easy and should be done routinely until familiarity with the terms is gained:

$$\text{Annual Simple Interest Rate} = \frac{\text{Trade Discount}}{100\% - \text{Trade Discount}} \times \frac{365 \text{ Days}}{\text{Payment Period} - \text{Discount Period}}$$

If a nursing home is offered terms of 2/10, net 30 for food supplies the annual simple interest rate is:

$$\begin{aligned}
\text{ASIR} &= \frac{2\%}{100\% - 2\%} \times \frac{365}{30 \text{ days} - 10 \text{ days}} \\
&= 0.0204 \times 18.25 \\
&= .3723 \text{ or } 37\%
\end{aligned}$$

This is a very favorable interest rate and should clearly be taken advantage of to minimize interest expense.

INVENTORY AND ACCOUNTS RECEIVABLE FINANCING

Another area in managing current liabilities is financing from inventory and accounts receivable. It is apparent that accounts receivable represent an asset (not a liability) that can be used to finance current operations. In this sense, accounts receivable can be used to finance current liabilities. Receivables represent an asset with substantial value. Although a health care organization does want to avoid using its receivables in this manner, there are extenuating circumstances that recommend that receivables be used to pay current liabilities. The strongest argument is when the receivables themselves have caused the liabilities but there is an unanticipated delay or shortfall in the receivables.

Inventory offers another convenient form of financing to meet current liabilities. Health care organizations have the advantage of extensive inventory of equipment and the disadvantage of perishable medical goods such as pharmaceuticals. Overall inventory cannot be used as extensively as it is in some business corporations due to the ephemeral quality of the goods.[28] However, exceptions can be found, particularly for multi-institutional systems with centralized purchasing where the value of the inventory is very high.

NOTES

1. Richard J. Oszustowicz, "Working Capital Management: How Strong Is It in Hospitals?" *Hospital Financial Management* 34 (April 1980): 12–20.
2. American Hospital Association, *Guidelines: Development of the Operating Margin* (Chicago, Ill.: AHA, Catalog No. G042, 1979), p. 1.
3. Frederick D. Margrif, "Short-term Cash Management for Hospitals," *Hospital Topics* 58 (September/October 1980): 8–9, 23.

4. Dave Person, "Payment Patterns," *Hospital Financial Management* 32 (June 1978): 36.
5. Robert M. Gottshall, "Condensed Control Reporting for Better Department Management," *Hospital Financial Management* 34 (June 1980): 64–67.
6. Robert L. Paretta and Robert J. Lipstein, "Internal Control: How Do Hospitals and Industry Compare?" *Hospital Financial Management* 33 (June 1979): 50–52.
7. Patrick Howard, Dirk N. Voetberg, and Allwyn J. Baptist, "Measurement, Feedback and Control: A Framework for Hospital Cost Containment," *Healthcare Financial Management* 38 (October 1984): 20–24.
8. G.W. Tonkin, "Cash: Stimulating the Flow," *Hospital Financial Management* 28 (August 1974): 22–30.
9. Crawford R. Hardy, "What Makes for Good Cash Management?" *Hospital Financial Management* 24 (April 1970): 24–27, 42.
10. Rodney Johnson, "Managing Your Working Capital: 2. Cash Discounts," *Hospital Financial Management* 29 (March 1975): 60–62.
11. Frederick D. Margrif, "Determining Excess Funds on a Daily Basis," *Hospital Financial Management* 35 (March 1981): 44–47.
12. Robert W. Broyles, *The Management of Working Capital in Hospitals* (Rockville, Md.: Aspen Publishers, 1981) pp. 172–173.
13. Lawrence D. Schall and Charles W. Haley, *Financial Management* (New York: McGraw-Hill, 1983) pp. 528–529.
14. Floyd A. Kinkead, "How to Use Reports to Gather Data for Better Management," *Hospital Financial Management* 29 (April 1975): 54–56.
15. Charles K. Bradford, "Bad Debts Are an Operating Expense," *Hospital Financial Management* 34 (February 1980): 49–51.
16. "Accounts Receivable Management—An Overview," *Topics in Health Care Financing* 8 (Spring 1982): 1–15.
17. Robert J. Kenneth and Gary L. Lampi, "The Management of Accounts Receivable," *Hospital Forum,* (February 1974): 9–11.
18. George P. Purvis, "How's Your Cash Flow?" *Hospital Financial Management* 30 (January 1976): 40–42.
19. Nancy J. Higgerson and Ann Van Slyck, "Variable Billing for Services: New Fiscal Direction for Nursing," *Journal of Nursing Administration* 12 (June 1982): 20–27.
20. Robert C. Bohlmann, "Profit Center Reporting—Made Easy," *Medical Group Management* 24 (November/December 1977): 38–41.
21. Philip Jacobs and Charles R. Franz, "Developing Pricing Policies by Diagnostic Grouping," *Healthcare Financial Management* 39 (January 1985): 50–52.
22. Clyde Goodbar, "Collections: Improving the Self-pay Balance Picture," *Hospital Financial Management* 35 (December 1981): 34–36.
23. "Control Receivable Days through Cross Training," *Healthcare Financial Management* 39 (March 1985): 93–94.
24. Richard A. Reid and William Koch, "Using Lock Boxes to Reduce Float Time," *Hospital Financial Management* 35 (December 1981): 38–43.
25. Robert A. Cerrone and Thomas Reca, "Periodic Interim Payments," in W.O. Cleverley, ed., *Handbook of Health Care Accounting and Finance* (Rockville, Md.: Aspen Publishers, 1982) pp. 1249–1269.

26. Cal Calhoun, "How to Eliminate Wide Swings in Monthly Income," *Hospital Financial Management* 35 (August 1981): 38–39, 42.

27. Bruce Fisher, "Patient Refunds and Credits Needn't Be a Pain," *Hospital Financial Management* 34 (December 1980): 28–29, 30–34.

28. Rodney Johnson, "Simulation: An Alternative Approach to Inventory Control," *Hospital Financial Management* 29 (July 1975): 48–53.

Chapter 7

Managing Costs

Nurse administrators have a high degree of sensitivity to the need for cost control. They are generally inundated with requests, policies, and programs from top management that are designed to hold down costs. Nurse administrators are central to these plans because nursing services represent a significant proportion of most costs in a health care organization. Additionally, nurses have many opportunities to influence costs not only in their practice, but also in the guidance they provide to personnel. For these reasons it is essential that nurse administrators clearly understand how costs behave, how nursing costs fit within the total spectrum of organizational costs, and how a knowledge of standard costs can ultimately lead to an effective management control system.

The specific skills in managing costs that are needed by nurse administrators vary considerably. In some cases a nurse administrator may wish only to become familiar with general costing procedures in order to understand and communicate better in the budgeting phase.[1] In other cases nurse administrators will be directly involved with the calculation and justification of costs or the preparation of reports and periodic budgets. In still other situations the nurse administrator will not only need an understanding of costs, but will also be responsible for analytically ascertaining costs (e.g., in a labor and delivery unit[2]), for justifying pricing decisions based on cost,[3] for participating in the budgeting process, or for commenting on a proposed program or service (e.g., all–registered nurse staffing[4]). The following material is designed to provide a general orientation to costs. The nurse administrator who discovers that job responsibilities entail specialization in cost accounting is advised to seek additional preparation in order to manage at the highest possible level of effectiveness.

DEFINITION OF COSTS

The accounting, finance, and economic disciplines are based equally on the concept of costs and cost behavior. Nurse administrators must be able to think and

177

speak fluently in this terminology if they expect to communicate effectively with other managers and with their staff members. Nurse administrators are responsible for translating budgets and plans into specific operational schedules and decisions. Even though it is vitally important to be able to converse with other managers, it is equally important that the issues surrounding costs be interpreted in a manner that is understandable by subordinates. Therefore, if the chief financial officer elicits an agreement from all nursing administrators to work on containing fixed costs, they must also be able to explain this in a nontechnical manner to their subordinates.

Direct and Indirect Costs

Nurse administrators should be capable of differentiating between direct and indirect costs. Direct costs are those that can be identified with and that result from the production of a specific good or the delivery of a specific service. There are many direct costs in any nursing program, but usually these costs are exemplified by the salaries of nurses, supplies used to provide services, and other costs that are germane to the specific clinical specialty. For example, in a urology ward, the direct nursing costs would include the salaries of the nursing team; the catheters, bandages, and pharmaceutical supplies used in treating patients; and possibly the costs of equipment depreciation for the ward itself (although under some accounting systems such costs may be viewed as indirect costs).

Indirect costs include costs that cannot be directly traced to a specific good or service, even though the indirect cost may be a necessary element in production of the good or delivery of the service. Utility costs are an excellent example of an indirect cost that must be used to produce nursing services but are not directly traceable to nursing services. A precise method for determining the amount of utilities consumed by a clinical nursing specialty would be installation of a computerized system of meters for monitoring the consumption of energy. Even with precise measurement, the specialty would use energy that should be assigned to the total organization because it achieves organizational rather than nursing unit goals. Since few health care organizations invest in such elaborate monitoring systems (due to the cost), an accounting convention is adopted that allocates utility costs on the basis of a common denominator, such as square footage.

Indirect costs should receive standard treatment from one period to the next if the organization intends to develop a precise cost accounting and allocation process. For this reason, indirect costs are standardized within most organizations. In the case of direct versus indirect costs, the issue is resolved in terms of the cost objective. A cost objective is the unit of production or service delivery that incurs the cost as part of its normal activities. For this reason, indirect costs can be allocated to any organizational unit or activity that incurs the cost in the production or service delivery process. In sum, there are generally accepted accounting principles that help distinguish between direct and indirect costs.

Examples of indirect costs generally include allocated costs from other departments (or overhead), costs of personnel administration, and depreciation. The nursing clinic in urology therefore may be assigned a proportion of indirect costs from the following support areas on this allocation basis:

- Food service (number of meals prepared)
- Depreciation (area in square feet)
- Medical records (number of patient days)
- Housekeeping (area in square feet)
- Administration (percentage of total costs)

Food service department costs would be allocated to the clinic on the basis of meals prepared for urology patients. Depreciation would be allocated according to the number of square feet in the clinic (relative to total square feet in the health care facility). Medical records costs are allocated as a proportion of patient days delivered by the clinic, compared with total patient days delivered by the organization. Housekeeping costs are allocated on the basis of square feet in the clinic. Administration is allocated according to the ratio of total nursing costs to total costs of the health care institution.

Note that whether a cost is defined as direct or indirect has little relation to whether the cost is viewed as fixed, variable, or semivariable. These terms are reserved to describe how certain costs fluctuate over time or for a given level of performance, not whether they are attached to a specific cost objective. This distinction is important to keep in mind. In the actual process of allocating costs, confusion can develop when a given cost is labeled in several different ways.

Allocable Costs

The difference between direct and indirect costs is important because of the principle of allocation. This concept is easy to forget when classifying costs, yet it has substantial practical implications. The allocation of costs is a process that can cause significant practical problems. Yet it is one that cannot be easily resolved even after the problem has been identified. Allocable costs represent an issue that every manager with budget responsibility should be vitally concerned about.

The issue of allocable costs involves how overhead or indirect costs are allocated to departments. As the discussion on indirect and direct costs suggested, there is a fundamental difference between costs that must be shared among productive units in an organization and costs that are directly attributed to a unit that produces a good or service. Indirect costs are generally defined as allocable costs that are divided among organizational units (both support and productive units) because it is difficult to identify the costs with any specific cost objective. These costs are allocated according to some rational basis of cost sharing. Direct costs, in contrast, are attributed to a specific cost objective or productive unit.

The problem between direct and indirect costs is not immediately apparent outside the budget process. A nurse administrator is responsible for keeping expenditures within budgeted targets. This is a reasonable assignment because of the delegation of authority to carry out this duty. If the nurse administrator needs to terminate a staff member, or implement stricter policies over inventory to ensure cost control, it can be accomplished due to the principle of delegated authority. In essence, the nurse administrator has direct control over the situation and may use whatever decision-making discretion is appropriate to achieve the desired results.

However, the nurse administrator will also discover that certain support, overhead, or indirect costs have been allocated to the nursing budget. This seems reasonable because any clinical nursing unit or nursing program is part of a larger organization. It must share in the burden of total costs incurred to support the main clinical services. What most managers overlook is that these so-called allocable costs are quite different from the direct costs that result from producing nursing services. The difference is profound, but there is no easy solution for the dilemma.

Careful thinking about indirect costs and direct costs shows that there is a distinct difference in the *ability to control* them. For direct costs, the nursing administrator is able to implement corrective actions to control costs when expenses exceed budgeted levels. The principle of delegated decision-making authority is applicable. For indirect costs, the nursing administrator confronts a serious predicament. Although the administrator has little or no control in how the support services are managed, the costs are nonetheless an integral part of a budget for which the administrator is responsible.

Assume that a nurse administrator has been successful in maintaining (i.e., with no increase) the direct costs of a clinic over three years. This administrator may still discover that the nursing budget has been exceeded if support services are ill managed or lack mechanisms and incentives for controlling costs. In essence, the nurse administrator can be held accountable for performance over which there was no control. By definition this violates the concept of management control.

For nurse administrators the problem of allocable costs is most apparent for support services such as housekeeping, food service, medical records, billing, administration, and operation of plant. It is not unusual to discover that a health care organization's cost containment program has been aimed at all of the main departments or functional areas, yet neglects the support services. On one hand there is a group of managers (i.e., in the main departments) doing everything possible to control the direct costs of their department or work unit, while on the other hand another group of managers (i.e., in support services) may be less involved in the cost control effort. Cost control is a matter of equal application of incentives, rewards, penalties, and ability to integrate units producing indirect costs with those consuming the services of support units.

Nurse administrators may discover that cost allocation discrimination exists in whole or in part for their organization. It is a serious problem that can be resolved when top management incorporates the support units on an equal basis in cost control. It makes little sense to have nursing doing everything possible to contain costs if housekeeping has no solid program for controlling its costs. In this case housekeeping is subsidized by the units producing direct costs. Therefore, the best advice for nurse administrators is to work with the financial staff in rectifying these anomalies when they occur.

Fixed Costs

Beyond the issue of where to assign specific costs, it is important to consider how costs behave over time. This so-called cost behavior acknowledges that changes in the amount of goods or services produced will influence the actual cost. There are four main types of cost behaviors including fixed, variable, semivariable, and step costs.[5] If the behavior patterns of costs are misinterpreted, it is possible to inadvertently err when preparing budgets.

In other situations mistakes will be made in assessing the feasibility of various programs (e.g., cost control[6]). For example, if the nurse administrator identifies the costs of processing data for billing as a fixed cost when in fact it is a step cost (i.e., decreases as increments of 1,000 bills are processed), then an incorrect budget has been predicted. Although this may not seem like an especially critical problem, the accumulation of unpredicted surpluses and deficits can lead to serious budgeting problems for the organization.

The first category of cost behavior is known as fixed costs. These costs do not vary with the volume of goods or services produced. Such a relationship between cost and volume can be depicted as follows:

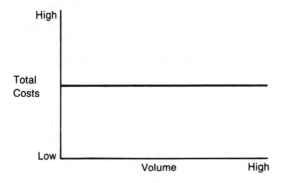

According to this depiction, total costs do not vary with volume. An illustration of this relationship is the principal and interest payment for a hospital mortgage. Each month the cost of the mortgage remains the same (assuming a fixed rate mortgage) despite the volume of patient days delivered. Therefore, if the hospital delivers 6,000 total days of inpatient care in April, the cost of the mortgage is equal to the cost in December when the hospital delivers only 4,500 days of inpatient care. The mortgage costs have not varied with the volume of services delivered, nor any other production or service function at the hospital. The mortgage costs are fixed at a single level.

What fixed costs normally occur in health care settings? Any cost that does not vary with respect to volume. These costs are usually centered around long-term investments in plant and major equipment that require an extensive length of time to pay off and for which a contractual agreement has been made to stabilize or fix payments. Depreciation costs—the inverse of capital investment—are also categorized as fixed costs because the amount of depreciation is often fixed over the life of the asset (e.g., ten years). The use of accelerated depreciation methods alters the fixed cost of depreciation, but careful reflection indicates that this is an accounting mechanism, not a cost behavior. Straight-line depreciation more accurately captures the life span and cost behavior of fixed assets.

Insurance on plant and equipment is another fixed cost in the health care setting. Although yearly insurance premiums may change, they do so without relation to volume. If a health institution rents or leases a facility or piece of equipment, these rent payments are also categorized as fixed costs. Remember that contracts vary, and it is not unusual to find a variable rate for such rental based upon use. For example, a photocopy machine may be rented for $743 per year. This is a fixed cost that can be spread out in monthly payments. The rental agency may charge another fee of $10 for every 1,000 copies exceeding 7,000 copies made per month. This additional fee is not a fixed cost, but a variable cost.

Nursing programs are very labor-intensive, and it is not surprising to find certain fixed labor costs. Usually these labor costs are fixed as a result of a contractual agreement. Therefore, when a nursing home enters into a contractual arrangement with a nursing registry to provide 40 hours of registered nursing care every month, it has incurred fixed costs. Whether volume of patient days goes up or down the cost of these nursing hours remains the same. In contrast the *total* nursing cost for this nursing home will go up as the number of patient days rises. Since licensure and third party payers require a certain level of skilled nursing hours served per patient day, the nursing home must either hire more staff nurses or agree to purchase more nursing hours from the registry.

These illustrations indicate another interesting feature of fixed costs. Although fixed costs do not vary according to volume, they do vary in relation to a specific level of units; that is, the unit cost will vary. If a food service department in a mental health center examines the cost of its major equipment it might find that it cost $18,000 for all fixed assets. These are fixed costs that depreciate at a methodical rate. However, the unit cost varies according to meals served. Assume a six-year life for the assets with straight-line depreciation.

Number of Meals Served	Depreciation Cost Per Meal Served
4,000	($18,000 ÷ 6) ÷ 4,000 = $0.75
5,000	($18,000 ÷ 6) ÷ 5,000 = $0.60
6,000	($18,000 ÷ 6) ÷ 6,000 = $0.50

The unit cost of depreciation is variable depending on the number of meals served. The cost may range from $.50 per meal at 6,000 meals to $.75 per meal when only 4,000 meals are served. Despite this unit variance in depreciation costs, the total depreciation costs are fixed. Higher or lower volume does not influence the total fixed costs—they remain the same.

Variable Costs

Variable costs are so named for their tendency to vary in relation to changes in volume. As the production of a good or service fluctuates so too will variable costs. The amount of variation may be direct or it may be proportional. Therefore, a direct variation of 20 percent more inpatient days served by a health maintenance organization should result in 20 percent more skilled and licensed practical nursing costs. This is a direct variation.

However, assume that the added nursing hours actually cost more per hour because the health maintenance organization has to retain part-time nurses. These nurses are less productive because they are assigned to different clinical specialties. Consequently they are unable to develop familiarity with other staff members or the policies, procedures, and regimens of each clinical unit. They are not as efficient because they spend more time trying to learn a unique process of care. Since the nurses are less productive, the health maintenance organization must acquire proportionately more nursing hours per increase in inpatient days served. Perhaps it requires 30 percent more skilled and licensed practical nursing hours (and hence costs) when there are 20 percent more inpatient days served. This is a proportional variation.

The relationship between cost and volume under variable costs is often very complex and difficult to specify because seldom do the relationships remain strictly direct or strictly proportional. Nurse administrators should recognize this fact and tolerate the inability to determine the cost–volume relationship precisely. What is needed is a useful approximation in order to forecast costs and then to formulate budgets. Nonetheless, it is critical to capture the variance in as precise a manner as possible in order to ensure the accuracy of these budgets.

The behavior of variable costs can be depicted as follows:

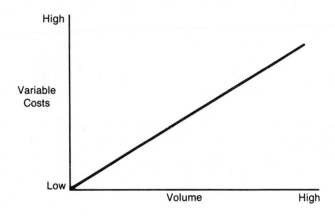

According to this diagram, as the volume of goods or services produced increases, so too do the total amount of costs. An illustration of their relationship is found in nursing supplies for a cardiac care unit. As the number of patients served per month increases 15 percent, the amount expended on supplies also increases 15 percent. If the number of patients served per month in June was the same as the number of patients served in July, then there would be no increase.

There are many examples of variable costs in the health care field. The amount of supplies consumed is a good example of variable costs because supply use is related to services delivered. Although there may not be a direct relationship due to the problem of case mix severity, supplies are generally consumed at a higher rate when the number of patients served increases. Labor costs represent another excellent example of variable costs. As more nurses are hired to cover the shifts in a hospital, the total costs of care also rise. Furthermore the employee benefits that accompany the cost of hiring the nurses also increases. Hence an increase in one cost area may produce other variable costs.

Like fixed costs, variable costs have a relationship to volume in the sense that volume affects either *total* fixed or *total* variable costs. When accounting for the impact on per unit of volume produced or served the association varies between fixed and variable costs. Assume that a food service department in a mental health center has been examining the cost of meals served over the last quarter. It discovers that it has incurred monthly total food costs of $4,000, $5,000 and $6,000. These figures represent the actual supplies used to produce the meals. In order to determine the cost per meal, the total food costs must be associated with the number of meals provided.

Total Monthly Food Cost	Total Meals Served	Cost per Meal
$4,000	3,200	$1.25
$5,000	4,000	$1.25
$6,000	4,800	$1.25

This analysis shows that the cost per meal for food supplies is a constant figure of $1.25. Thus, *total* food costs are a variable cost that will vary according to the number of meals served and hence food supplies consumed.

It is useful to observe the distinction between fixed costs and variable costs in the variance for the cost per unit. Fixed costs may vary for each unit but will remain fixed in total amount. In other words, the cost of nursing equipment per patient day will be different in a given month if there are 1,000 patients compared with 1,500 patients. But the *total* cost of the nursing equipment remains the same in each month regardless of changes in number of patients served.

For variable costs, the relationship is reversed. The total costs will vary while the cost per unit will remain the same. For example, the cost of nursing supplies per patient will be $5.76 whether there are 1,000 or 1,500 patients. The total cost of the nursing supplies will vary respectively, in this instance, from $5,760 to $8,640 for these patient totals. The point is that the unit cost and total cost capture the difference between fixed and variable costs.

Semivariable Costs

Nurse administrators may conclude that costs are seldom as well defined as being either fixed or variable costs. Reality indicates that costs often fall between these two categories. At some point a cost may take on the qualities of fixed costs; in other instances it behaves like a variable cost. Because of this fluctuation, nurse administrators should be familiar with semivariable costs. Some production or service activities will produce costs that generally vary with volume but at other times are fixed. In other cases they vary at a rate different than that associated with volume. In short, semivariable costs have both fixed and variable components.

A good illustration of semivariable costs in the health care field is found in the costs of maintaining expensive pieces of diagnostic and therapeutic equipment. When this equipment is new, the cost of maintaining it is relatively fixed per year. However, as the equipment ages or begins to require more adjustments, repairs, and preventive attention, variability enters into the picture of cost behavior. The equipment may require steadily increasing investments in order to remain operable. The extent of use can exacerbate this situation. Greater use will result in more rapid deterioration of the equipment. Hence, in a year of particularly heavy use, the cost of maintenance may rise higher than at other points in time. These trends are depicted in the following example of a magnetic resonance imager as:

Age of Equipment	Number of Scans	Repair Costs	General Maintenance Costs	Total Costs
1	900	$ 0	$1,200	$1,200
2	950	$ 0	$1,200	$1,200
3	1,400	$3,345	$1,200	$4,545
4	1,000	$ 500	$1,200	$1,700
5	1,200	$1,000	$1,200	$2,200

The total maintenance costs vary from $1,200 to $4,545 per year.

The semivariable costs for maintaining the magnetic resonance imager comprise both fixed costs (i.e., $1,200 routine monthly maintenance) and variable costs (i.e., costs for repair, such as $500 in year 4). The problem for the health care manager is to estimate the variable portion of the cost of maintenance. Although this is a difficult process, it must be done in order to arrive at some understanding of how costs will behave over the next operating period. A budget must be based upon these estimates. In some situations this estimation is relatively easy because the equipment has been used for a long period of time and costs can be anticipated. In the case of substantially new technology the estimate may be more a guess than a rational calculation.

Semivariable costs can be depicted:

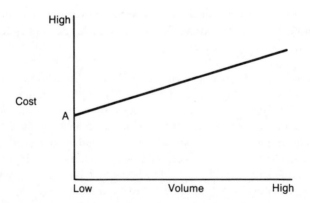

In this graph the semivariable cost includes a fixed component (perhaps a yearly rent) that is denoted by point A. As volume increases, the total costs also increase. In the case of the magnetic resonance imager, the variable costs of maintenance fluctuated from $0 to $3,345, while volume varied from 900 to 1,400 scans. An approximation of the yearly variable cost portion of maintaining the equipment is equal to:

$$\frac{\text{Total Variable Costs}}{\text{Total Number of Scans}} = \text{Average yearly variable cost per scan}$$

$$\frac{(\$0 + 0 + 3,345 + 500 + 1,000)}{(\$900 + 950 + 1,400 + 1,000 + 1,200)} = \frac{\$4,845}{5450} = \$.89$$

According to this estimate, every scan results in an additional cost of $.89 of variable cost. The fixed portion is estimated as:

$$\frac{\text{Total Fixed Costs}}{\text{Total Number of Scans}} = \text{Average yearly fixed costs per scan}$$

$$\frac{(1,200 \times 5)}{5450} = \$1.10$$

Therefore the total semivariable costs of maintaining the imager are $.89 + $1.10 = $1.99 per scan.

Step Costs

The fourth type of cost behavior is known as step costs. It is a form of variable cost since it is not fixed. This cost is also termed a semifixed cost because at certain volume levels the cost does not vary. This mix of fixed and variable cost behavior is different from the semivariable cost in that the cost may be fixed over wide variances in volume. The following graph distinguishes step costs from semivariable costs in the sense of variable and fixed portions:

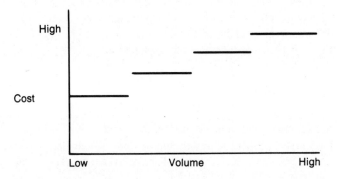

Note that the cost remains fixed for various volume levels and then it increases, only to remain at the fixed level over another volume increment before the process repeats itself.

Nurse administrators encounter many situations where step costs are involved. Perhaps the most immediately recognizable situation involves staff salaries. When a nursing unit has four staff nurses the salaries are fixed relative to the volume of patient care delivered. If there are few patients, the nurses' salaries still must be paid at the same amount as though there were many patients. Assume that the number of patients served begins to exceed the capacity of the nursing unit to deliver a proper standard of care. In this situation another nurse must be added to the unit to make a total of five nurses. However, if there is only one patient served by the nurse, the unit still must pay the salaries of five nurses. If there are 100 more patients served, the unit also must pay the salaries of five nurses. At some point the number of patients served again exceeds the service capacity of the nursing unit and another staff nurse must be added. This steps up the cost by another salary increment.

In health care organizations step costs are often the most prevalent cost because volume dictates resource investment. When hospital occupancy rises, nursing staff salaries increase, but so do all of the associated salary/wage costs in the support services. Once a hospital has hired new staff members its employee benefits costs will also increase. In line with these increases come higher expenses for administration. Higher occupancy implies a need for more supplies to treat and diagnose illness. There will also be higher supply costs in the support areas such as housekeeping, food service, and maintenance. Higher utility costs will also be experienced.

The profile that emerges is one that initially appears controllable, but actually health care managers are confronted with a dilemma. On one hand they must provide for the appropriate needs of patient demand, but on the other hand they need to contain those costs associated with providing the higher level of services. Since many of these costs are step costs, it is critical that nurse administrators and other financially responsible managers operate at the end of the step cost margin; that is, operations should be oriented toward maximizing return from resources. This means that judicious assessments must be made of the need to add resources, since each addition is a step up in costs. Demand must be present to justify fixed increments in costs that will occur in these situations.

CALCULATING COSTS AND COST BEHAVIOR

Now that a foundation has been set for understanding cost behavior, the nurse administrator is still confronted by a problem of how to calculate costs and how to predict in what manner these costs will behave over time. This is an especially difficult problem that is more deceptive than it appears at first glance. The reason is that there is a proliferation of cost centers within the typical health care organization.[7] This is complicated by the desire of management to maximize the reimbursement obtained from third party payers. As a result, the typical health care organization has an oversupply of cost reports and accounting systems. There are reports on virtually everything, but seldom is there the proper information needed to make decisions. This fact is particularly true for nurse administrators who are responsible for ascertaining the costs of their department, yet who may have little control over the standardized reports used in an organization.

These problems in costing-out aspects of nursing programs are very serious, because without reliable cost estimates it is difficult to justify requests for more resources, and it is difficult to document good performance. As a result of these problems there has been growing interest in developing standard cost systems.[8] A preliminary step to the formulation of standard costs is to calculate or estimate the behavior of costs involved in a given product or service area.

The problem in calculating cost behavior is essentially one of calculating costs themselves. Remember that the accounting records of a health care organization are excellent at depicting broad categories of costs, but they are not very successful in determining specifics about costs. For example, it is easy to determine how much nursing staff time costs in a given clinical specialty such as pediatrics. In contrast it is very difficult to determine the exact cost of the nursing time that went into caring for patients with broken limbs. The accounting records will convey the costs for nurse staffing and for supplies, but there will be no entries for the specific service.

Nurse administrators are increasingly being called upon to determine the exact cost of services delivered in nursing units. As a result, many have had to turn to cost accounting and operations management techniques in order to derive a satisfactory estimate that can serve as a basis for planning and decision making. These estimates are used when there is no previous record (or analysis) of the costs, or where it is difficult to readily identify cost patterns. Obviously if such patterns are impossible to discern it will also be extremely difficult to judge whether costs are direct or indirect, and whether they can be categorized as fixed, variable, semivariable, or step costs.

Operations management employs the scientific method to observe and document the process of providing nursing services. It is an effort to determine relationships between actions (or investments of resources) and outcomes. Therefore operations analysis can be employed to determine the level of costs that surround a parent education program staffed by nurses. Perhaps the director of nursing wishes to estimate the added cost of doubling the number of classes offered. How much will it cost and how will the specific costs behave? The answer to these questions can be derived from cost accounting, operations management, systems analysis, or industrial engineering methods when the information is not readily available from the traditional accounting system:

- Break down the organization of the parent education program into readily identifiable activities of a similar nature (e.g., classroom teaching, counseling, and administration).
- Sample the allocation of time devoted to each activity over the course of one month.
- Determine the amount of supplies used by monitoring the distribution of materials to parents and other individuals, agencies, or organizations demanding services.
- Analyze accounting records to determine specific dollar costs for supplies and nursing staff.
- Calculate a standard cost for nursing staff time (e.g., 25 percent of monthly salary for classroom teaching, 25 percent for counseling, and 50 percent for administration).
- Calculate a standard cost for supplies used (e.g., 10 percent of total supplies for classroom teaching, 5 percent for counseling, and 5 percent for administration).
- Analyze accounting records to determine the specific dollar costs for overhead. Distribute the overhead equally among the activity areas.

Admittedly this illustration is only a beginning of cost analysis, but the purpose is to demonstrate how *analysis* can be used to supplement rather sketchy information contained in the accounting system. A more rational basis is developed for planning, especially in the area of estimating specific costs and how they are predicted to behave.

Many analytical methods for calculating costs and cost behavior have been used in business and in the public sector. Increasingly these methodologies are being applied to health care organizations as managers demand more precise cost information for improving decision making. Some of these techniques include:

- jury of executive or managerial opinion (to estimate costs)
- systems analysis
- operations analysis
- multivariate analysis
- management science
- industrial engineering
- correlational analysis

There are many other techniques available which are not only useful for identifying cost elements for specific tasks, they are also useful for establishing a basis from which operations can be improved.

It is critical to understand fully where these analytical techniques can be used to estimate costs and cost behavior in health care settings. Some examples include ascertaining the costs of inventory (e.g., the cost of breakage, storage, and accident costs in using glass storage bottles versus plastic storage bottles), required transactions to complete a medical record, specific resources allocated to a nursing unit (e.g., personnel by type, supplies, overhead, and so forth), steps in the billing process, administrative support (e.g., computerized information systems support, management time for planning various aspects of operations, etc.), and job analysis of support personnel who supplement a nursing unit. These are only a few of the situations in which analysis can be used to estimate cost parameters. Nurse administrators must recognize that it is important to selectively analyze costs with the intention of improving plans (e.g., budgets) or decisions.

DETERMINING STANDARD COSTS

For several reasons it is becoming increasingly important for nurse administrators to undertake cost analysis. First, there is the issue of budgeting. In order for nursing units to develop sound estimates of programmatic costs it is vital that a valid cost profile be developed. Large health care organizations are increasingly creating staff positions (often filled by nurses with financial training or experience) to attend to the budgetary aspects of nursing departments. Fundamental to the sound completion of this responsibility is a knowledge of how costs behave and how to calculate a standard cost estimate for specific nursing activities. It is very difficult to create a realistic budget unless there is some rational basis for estimating the cost of specific resource inputs.

Second, nursing must reach a point where it is able to define precisely how much it will cost to provide services. At issue here is the need to justify resource allocations. Since nursing is basically a labor–intensive service, and since with prospective payment health care facilities are interested in cutting costs wherever they can, nursing is often targeted for these budget cuts. Through such reductions a health care organization is able to save substantial fixed and variable costs not only in employee salaries and benefits, but also in the resources needed to support nursing activities. This may seem to be logical behavior on the part of a hospital or nursing home, but at the nursing level where there is reduced staffing such resource cuts are experienced in their fullest. Ultimately it is the staff nurse who must be productive because staffing has been reduced. From the perspective of economic theory this may seem ideal (to the organization), but to the individual nurse who is making sacrifices the request can have a serious impact on morale.

The nurse administrator must be convincing when communicating the fact that additional resources are needed or justified. Usually it is the chief executive officer or the chief financial officer who need to be convinced that a nursing unit, program, or department deserves additional funds. In large hospitals or other health care facilities that are staffed intensively with nurses it is increasingly common to adopt sophisticated scheduling models in order to reduce the slack time available in nursing hours. These cost control efforts have the effect of considering cost and nursing hours first and other relevant considerations second. It is critical for health care organizations to move toward emphasis on cost control, but it is also important for them to dispense budget reductions equitably.

Since nursing programs are often the first to be targeted for reductions, it is imperative that nurse administrators be capable of documenting the need for resources (whether nursing hours, supplies, facilities, equipment, or support help) and justifying their arguments. The starting point for such activity is to establish a base estimate of costs and their behavior. This approach is known as the standard cost system. It has its origins in cost accounting and industrial engineering, where analysis of costs is a prelude to budgetary formulations.

Suver and Neumann as well as other authorities in the area suggest that there are several key steps for a standard cost system:[9,10]

- Analyze accounting records and charts of accounts to ascertain the specific categories of expenses and how they have varied over time (i.e., undertake historical cost analysis).
- Determine for these expenses the typical variations that these costs undergo in terms of seasonal fluctuation and volume variations.
- Classify the costs into specific behavior types—fixed, variable, semivariable, and semifixed.
- Analyze the unit of measure in order to derive as accurate a profile of basic activities as possible (e.g., nursing time devoted to patient care, administration of nurses, administration of programmatic activities, administration of organizational requirements, and so forth).
- Predict possible fluctuations in volume (e.g., high, medium, and low demand; 5 percent, 10 percent, and 15 percent increases on a base volume prediction).
- Predict resource investments according to the unique alternative profiles of staffing levels.
- Accumulate projections per standard costs.

The goal of the standard cost format is to improve the accuracy of predicting costs per level of activity. Although the standard costs are formulated on the basis of analysis of accounting records and application of more sophisticated quantitative techniques, there is still sufficient room for error in the ultimate formulation of cost profiles. Nonetheless it is this sort of *analytical* cost projection that helps improve the accuracy of budgets and the ultimate allocation of resources in health care organizations.

An example of the standard cost system is readily seen in the staffing problems of a geriatric nursing clinic. Table 7–1 provides an estimate of the standard costs for running such a program.

As the illustration in Table 7–1 indicates, the standard cost per patient treated in the clinic is $10.25. This cost incorporates both fixed and variable costs. It is assumed to be a perfectly variable cost in this example because the number of nurse practitioners in the clinic will be only two. Hence it is unlikely that there will be great variation in demand for overhead or supplies. Remember that if there were a significant fluctuation in demand or patients served, then it is possible that the cost projections for the overhead or supplies would be altered.[11] This is due to their variable and semivariable nature. As more and more supplies were consumed there would be a greater potential for reductions in the cost per unit of supply. Presumably the director of purchasing and materials management would be able to negotiate a lower rate for the supplies due to higher bulk purchases.

Table 7–1 Standard Cost for Geriatric Nursing Clinic

Assumptions	
Nursing Costs per Hour	$ 17.30
(for one geriatric nurse practitioner)	
Number of Patients Served per Hour	4
Cost of Supplies Consumed per Patient	$ 2.12
Departmental Overhead per Day	$120.76
Estimated Number of Nurse Practitioners	2
Working in the Unit Over the Entire Year	

Calculation of Standard Cost per Patient		
Nursing Staff Time	= $17.30 ÷ 4	= $ 4.35
Supplies Cost	=	$ 2.12
Departmental Overhead	= $120.76 ÷ (4 × 8)	= $ 3.78
Cost per Patient		$10.25

Calculation of Standard Hourly Costs For a Program Incorporating 2 Nurse Practitioners
Hourly Costs = 2 practitioners × 4 patients × $10.25 = $82.00

The power of calculating a standard cost for the geriatric nursing clinic is the ability to link the budget with costs and demand. As Table 7–1 indicates, if two nurse practitioners are working at capacity in the clinic the total cost would be $82.00 per hour for serving eight patients. With this information, the nurse administrator is able to project a yearly cost based on the assumptions in the example. This is a valuable aspect of the standard cost system, but it is not the only meaningful benefit. The nurse administrator is also in a position to predict the consequences of altering the rate of productivity.

Assume that the nurse administrator is concerned with raising the productivity of each nurse practitioner to five patients per hour. All of the needed information is available to estimate the impact of a change in productivity. This estimate must recognize that certain incentives will have to be given to the nurses to encourage an increase in productivity of 25 percent. Very likely this incentive could be added compensation or a bonus tied to the ability to meet a production goal. Once this estimated cost is forecasted it will be necessary to adjust the standard costs accordingly. It is entirely possible that no incentive will be awarded. As many nurse administrators recognize, health care organizations are demanding higher productivity from employees without generally providing commensurate increases. Therefore, it is possible that the standard costs will remain as calculated in Table 7–1 except for alteration because of the productivity increase.

In addition to the many benefits of using standard costs illustrated in the geriatric clinic, it is essential that nurse administrators also remain aware of the usefulness of standard costs in calculating prices. There was a tendency in the past for health care organizations to utilize rather gross methods for determining prices or charges. Usually rates were set after examining forecasted expenses and comparing these to forecasted demand at given rates. This process is still legitimate; however, the availability of the standard cost system allows greater accuracy in forecasting expenses and prices, especially as related to nursing standards.[12]

When setting rates it is essential that a comprehensive system of standard costs be available in order to precisely determine the overall cost of services. Note that even with the most careful and calculated effort at ascertaining standard costs there is still room for substantial error in the budget. This error enters into the calculations in the sense of forecasted patient demand. Despite sophisticated computer assistance, it is still difficult to correctly forecast the level of demand possible for given clinical services. The result is that determining charges—to cover the estimated expenses plus buffers for contingencies and a return on investment—may be inaccurate despite the best efforts at attaining precision. Such is the nature of forecasting and rate setting.

Variance Analysis

Once a health care organization has managed to develop an operationally effective program for budgeting and controlling costs, there is the problem of determining how to fine-tune operations. Generally this focus comes after the organization has established a working basis for estimating costs and their behaviors and for creating a profile of standard costs. Attention is devoted to determining how to make services more profitable or how to create better performance. This analysis is facilitated by the framework in which costs can be carefully examined and deviances resolved. For nurse administrators these efforts typically involve observing trends in standard costs or in productivity. Once deviances are identified, it is much easier to resolve a specific problem because attention is centered on the factors that ultimately result in higher or lower costs.

Nurse administrators should recognize that performance can almost always be improved. Staff productivity can be raised, or costs can be contained. These gains are possible once methodical analysis has validated that a problem does in fact exist. The challenge for nurse administrators is to create a monitoring system that identifies these deviations. While analysis of operations is healthy, nurse administrators must avoid developing a system that makes them monitor operations more than they manage operations. If their control system requires excessive time in analyzing data they run the risk of misdirecting their managerial time.

Once problems have been detected, alternative strategies can be formulated for improving performance. The advantage of this approach is that problem resolution builds on empirically articulated problems.[13,14] The problems are essentially variances in cost or productivity that need to be brought under control. This is where the concept of cost variance originates. The nurse administrator is responsible for knowing when a variance occurs and how to rectify the situation. For example, the nurse administrator of a triage team in an urban health center's outpatient clinic may spend considerable time defining standard costs and productivity for the registered nurses on the unit. This baseline of costs and productivity is useful for assessing the progress made in the unit itself. The data act as a standard from which it is possible to pinpoint specific cost deviances or low output.

Preferably the cost and productivity baselines can be used to prevent deviances before they occur. This is direct control. It is predicated on the belief that the best way to manage a program is to prevent deviances, rather than to let operations run a complete course to the extent that problems occur. While this is undeniably the preferred state of affairs, the ability to actually implement such tight control in a nursing context is questionable. The nursing administrator may be unable to allocate substantial time to monitoring performance. Even if the nurse administrator were able to do this, there is a question whether such tight control is desirable. It is unlikely that professionals will enjoy such scrutiny.

Under most conditions, it is possible to implement periodic control over performance in both costs and productivity. Consequently, the feasibility of cost variance analysis is considerably improved. The main question becomes how to implement such a system. What steps are involved? How does it function? These questions depend on the specific nursing tasks involved, the availability of data, and the information needed to ascertain the direction of performance.

Consider the following performance data for a kidney dialysis treatment center in which cost and productivity variances have been monitored:

	Year 1	Year 2	Year 3
Number of FTE RNs	2	2.5	3.0
Average Yearly Salary (per RN)	$25,000	$26,500	$28,000
Supplies per Patient	$150	$160	$175
Number of Patients	360	380	410

It is possible to calculate the cost variance in the following fashion:

Cost of RN Staffing

(Year 1 to 2) = $26,500 − $25,000 = $1,500
(Year 2 to 3) = $28,000 − $26,500 = $1,500

Cost Variance of RN Staffing

(Year 1 to 2) = $1,500 × 2.5 FTE = $3,750
(Year 2 to 3) = $1,500 × 3.0 FTE = $4,500

The changes in cost variances resulting from alterations in staffing, and costs of staffing, can be determined. Clearly the cost variance of staffing between Years 1 and 2 versus the difference in Years 2 and 3 is much lower. This trend is obscured in the data unless a proportional difference is calculated. The data suggest that there is an increasing cost of registered nurse staffing (per full time equivalent) in the third year. The cost difference may or may not be important; what is critical is that by monitoring the staffing cost variances, the nurse administrator is alerted to a potentially negative trend. This is the contribution of analysis of cost variances to improved management. The nurse administrator is alerted to the deviance early enough that meaningful action can be implemented to prevent further escalation of costs.

Similarly it is possible to assess the variance in the supplies cost per patient. According to the data:

Cost of Supplies

(Year 1 to Year 2) = $160 − $150 = $10
(Year 2 to Year 3) = $175 − $160 = $15

Cost Variance of Supplies

(Year 1 to Year 2) = $10 × (380 − 360) = $200
(Year 2 to Year 3) = $15 × (410 − 380) = $450

This is a serious variance that deserves close scrutiny. The problem is that the cost variance in supplies is increasing at a rate faster than that noted for staffing. This means that careful attention should be paid to supplies costs in the forthcoming year. With investigative analysis, it may be possible to pinpoint the discrepancy (e.g., perhaps the added one-half time staff nurse has not been oriented to the supply practices and policies of the unit; the nurse may need a more thorough orientation).

As the preceding examples have suggested, the ability to analyze variances in cost and productivity are beneficial because it is then possible to address specific deviations. Although cost variance analysis does not totally explain why costs vary, it does provide information that points managers in the correct direction. The nurse administrator must complete this investigation by demanding further data, conducting additional analysis, or discussing the variances with the staff or other managers who might lend valuable guidance. Cost variance analysis is not the ultimate explanation for why costs have varied—it is only a prelude to further analysis from which more reliable answers can be determined.

NURSING COSTS BY ACUITY

The calculation of nursing costs has become steadily more complex in recent years. The introduction of relative intensity measures for nursing services under diagnosis related group (DRG) payment epitomizes the increasing sophistication needed to determine nursing costs.[15] Although there is ongoing disagreement about the precise method for estimating the amount of nursing services consumed within patient-specific case mix length of stay statistics in the DRG system, it is apparent that future payment systems will require estimation of nursing costs based around acuity.[16,17] The rationale behind these cost systems is that patient severity influences the amount of nursing services consumed. A high level of severity requires more nursing care than a low level of severity. Therefore, the cost is higher, which justifies a higher reimbursement level.

A related concern in the calculation of nursing costs under DRG systems is the extent to which DRG payments accurately reflect nursing resources consumed.[18] If the payments do not incorporate the true costs of nursing care, then it is possible that a hospital will be unable to derive a net operating margin over all DRGs. In view of this problem, hospitals and other health care organizations have substantial motivation to manage case mix information carefully and to use standard cost accounting.[19–21] These management practices must be applied to nursing programs and departments in order to calculate the relative contribution of nursing to costs and profits within each DRG.

Some analyses of nursing costs relative to total hospital charges have implied that nursing costs are but a small percentage of these total charges. One study at Stanford University Hospital in California suggests that nursing care costs are only 17.8 percent of total hospital charges (over six diagnoses) and actually range from

14 to 21 percent of total charges.[22] This finding was corroborated by a study at St. Paul-Ramsey Medical Center in Minnesota.[23] The conclusion of these studies is that nursing costs are a relatively minor component of total hospital charges. Yet they may overlook one important point. With tightening restrictions on reimbursement it is essential to control *all* costs regardless of proportional contribution to total costs. Thus nursing costs are an important element of total cost control, even though they may vary extensively according to diagnosis or acuity.[24]

Costing nursing services under diagnosis related reimbursement necessitates the inclusion of acuity level with normal cost estimations.[25,26] For example, assume that two nursing wards produced the following direct costs:

	Census	Nursing Hours per Day	Total Hours	Total Direct Nursing Costs	Average Cost per Nursing Hour
Ward 1	100	6.00	600	$10,050	$16.75
Ward 2	250	3.40	850	$12,750	$15.00

The units experienced the following variances in acuity:

	Acuity Level	Patient %	Patient #	Hours of Care per Level	Total Hours per Level	Direct Cost per Level	Direct Cost per Level per Patient
Ward 1	Level II	83	83	4.80	398.4	$6,673.20	$ 80.40
	Level III	17	17	11.86	201.6	3,376.80	198.64
Ward 2	Level I	54	135	2.79	307.6	5,649.00	41.84
	Level II	46	115	4.20	483.0	7,245.00	63.00

By determining:

1. the average cost per nursing hour,
2. the dispersion of patients according to acuity level, and
3. the average number of hours of care per level

it is possible to ascertain the direct cost per acuity level by multiplying the total hours per acuity level by the average cost per nursing hour. This yields the direct cost per level per patient. The calculation of the *total* nursing cost by patient acuity level then depends on the allocation of indirect costs. For example:

	Acuity Level	Nursing Cost per Patient	Hospital and Nursing Administration Costs per Patient	Support Services Cost per Patient	Total Cost per Patient
Ward I	Level II	$ 80.04	$20.00	$ 62.10	$162.14
	Level III	198.64	25.00	110.00	333.64
Ward II	Level I	41.84	21.00	54.44	117.28
	Level II	63.00	20.00	39.13	122.13

By calculating the total nursing cost per patient according to acuity level it is possible to formulate more accurate nursing budgets. For nursing this implies that a more equitable allocation of resources will be provided that is consistent with patient service needs.

The preparation of nursing budgets is contingent on information systems that provide accurate data on costs. Before the concept of acuity can be used to modify the nursing cost per patient day it is essential that the information system be upgraded to reflect the best calculations and estimates of direct and indirect costs. Until this is achieved it will be difficult to undertake budget modifications based on patient acuity.

NOTES

1. Eduard Marenco, "Accounting Concepts and Techniques for Managing Continuing Education and Inservice," *Nursing Administration Quarterly* 3 (Fall 1978): 75–81.

2. Jeanne Flyntz De Joseph, Barbara J. Petrie, and William Ross, "Costing and Charging: Pricing care in OB," *Nursing Management* 15 (December 1984): 36–37.

3. Donald F. Beck, "Health Care Financial Management: General concepts for the Hospital Pharmacist," *Topics in Hospital Pharmacy* 10 (Spring 1984): 66–76.

4. Ada Sue Hinshaw, Robert Scofield, and Jan R. Atwood, "Staff, Patient, and Cost Outcomes of All–Registered Nurse Staffing," *Journal of Nursing Administration* 11 (November/December 1981): 30–36.

5. Joseph E. Nagy, "To Reduce Costs Hospitals Must Identify Fixed and Variable Costs," *Hospital Financial Management* 36 (March 1982): 50–54.

6. Paul Slowiak, "How Department Heads Can Use Cost Studies to Reduce Hospital Costs," *Hospital Topics* 62 (November/December 1984): 26–27.

7. William J. Riley and Vicki Schaefers, "Nursing Operations as a Profit Center," *Nursing Management* 15 (April 1984): 43–46.

8. Wayne M. Lerner, William L. Wellman, and David Burik, "Pricing of Hospital Units of Service Using Microcosting Techniques," *Hospital and Health Services Administration* 30 (January/February 1985): 7–28.

9. James D. Suver and Bruce R. Neumann, "Standard Costs for Healthcare Providers," *Hospital Financial Management* 35 (February 1981): 32–34, 36.

10. David Burik and Thomas J. Duvall, "Hospital Cost Accounting: A Basic System Framework," *Healthcare Financial Management* 39 (March 1985): 58–64.

11. Frances M. Hoffman, "Cost per RN Hired," *Journal of Nursing Administration* 15 (February 1985): 27–29.

12. Elizabeth J. Mason and Judith K. Daugherty, "Nursing Standards Should Determine Nursing's Price," *Nursing Management* 15 (September 1984): 34–38.

13. Anthony Wellever, "Variance Analysis: A Tool for Cost Control," *Journal of Nursing Administration* 12 (July/August 1982): 23–26.

14. Werner G. Frank, "A Managerial Accounting Analysis of Hospital Costs," *Health Services Research* 11 (Spring 1976): 34–44.

15. Russell P. Caterinicchio, "Relative Intensity Measures: Pricing of Inpatient Nursing Services under Diagnosis-related Group Prospective Hospital Payment," *Health Care Financing Review* 6 (Fall 1984): 61–70.

16. Russell P. Caterinicchio, "A Defense of the RIMs Study," *Nursing Management* 14 (May 1983): 36–39.

17. P.L. Grimaldi and Julie A. Micheletti, "A Defense of the RIMs Critique—RIMs Reliability and Value?" *Nursing Management* 14 (May 1983): 40–41.

18. Malinda Mitchell et al., "Determining Cost of Direct Nursing Care by DRGs," *Nursing Management* 15 (April 1984): 43–46.

19. Marilyn P. Plomann, Gerald E. Bisbee, and Truman Esmond, "Use of Case–Mix Information in Hospital Management: An Overview and Case Study," *Healthcare Financial Management* 38 (October 1984): 28–31, 34–36, 40–42.

20. Marilyn P. Plomann and Truman Esmond, "Using Case–Mix Information for Budgeting," *Healthcare Financial Management* 38 (October 1984): 30–31, 34–35.

21. Victor C. Messmer, "Methods That Can Be Applied to DRG Classifications," *Healthcare Financial Management* 38 (January 1984): 44–45, 48.

22. Duane D. Walker, "The Cost of Nursing Care in Hospitals," *Journal of Nursing Administration* 13 (March 1983): 13–18.

23. William Riley and Vicki Schaefers, "Costing Nursing Services," *Nursing Management* 14 (December 1983): 40–43.

24. Richard C. McKibbin et al., "Nursing Costs and DRG Payments," *American Journal of Nursing* (December 1985): 1353–1356.

25. Ann Butler Maher and Barbara Dolan, "Determining Cost of Nursing Services," *Nursing Management* 13 (September 1982) 17–21.

26. Pamela de Mars Martin and Frank J. Boyer, "Developing a Consistent Method for Costing Hospital Services," *Healthcare Financial Management* 39 (February 1985): 30–31, 34–37.

Chapter 8

Capital Budgeting and Analysis

Plant and equipment are essential to any health care organization. It is through the physical assets of the medical clinic, nursing home, or hospital that health care goods and services are produced. The trends toward decentralized service delivery and outpatient care may revolutionize the health care field, but they will not erase the need for a central capital asset base. Consequently, every health care organization must carefully replenish this base not only to remain operational but also to adjust to new competitive, technological, reimbursement, and economic pressures.

Nursing administrators must be sensitive to the changing uses of capital assets. They are responsible for managing the impact of capital investment decisions on current operations and on long-run nursing service delivery patterns. For example, innovations in outpatient clinics have caused considerable concern for nursing administrators. Emergency centers and urgent care clinics have given nurses additional opportunities aside from their traditional roles in large medical centers and hospitals. Often there are added responsibilities for managing facilities, equipment, and personnel. Furthermore, nursing administrators are confronting a raised financial consciousness. As a result, they may not be fully prepared to participate in planning for capital assets—their acquisition, use, and expansion.

The participation of nurse administrators in capital asset decisions and capital budgeting is consistent with established trends in business. There has been a growing commitment to decentralized capital budgeting in business organizations. Mid- and lower-level managers are increasingly being integrated into capital asset planning. Nursing administrators are experiencing this same phenomenon and will be involved more extensively in capital issues in the future. Therefore, nurse administrators need to be thoroughly grounded in capital asset budgeting to provide reasoned and meaningful input to this process.

CAPITAL BUDGETING AND TOTAL FINANCIAL OPERATIONS

Long-term assets invested in plant and major pieces of equipment are generally defined as capital assets. These fixed assets differ from current assets in that they

201

are not likely to be liquidated in less than one year. Minor pieces of equipment are sometimes viewed as current assets (as opposed to capital assets), depending on their total valuation and the length of time for their depreciation. The rapid obsolescence of some diagnostic and treatment equipment implies that it should be included in the current asset category, but the fact that this equipment may require substantial monetary investment generally limits it to the capital asset category.

Capital budgeting is the process of planning and decision making for capital assets. Among other main characteristics, capital budgeting involves:

- Determining the demand for services, which in turn has an impact on the need for expansion, addition, or improvement in physical plant and equipment
- Ascertaining the financial feasibility of expenditures on capital assets
- Calculating what level of expenditure on capital assets is possible, given total financial requirements and prevailing revenue streams
- Evaluating capital asset options for their ability to meet preestablished investment criteria
- Planning how capital expenditures will fit with the long-run financial plans of an institution

It is apparent that capital budgeting should be a continuous activity—it is not effectively conducted on an intermittent basis. Yet, this is precisely the point that is often overlooked by many health care managers.

Historical Trends Affecting Capital Budgeting

Capital budgeting within the context of total financial operations in the health care industsry has been particularly neglected. The reasons for this neglect are extensive, but they generally seem to have one commonality—third party reimbursement. After several decades of cost-pass-through reimbursement and government subsidizing of new facility construction, health care organizations became rather complacent about capital budgeting. Hospitals particularly depended on government grants and Hill-Burton funding that represented a convenient source of capital funds. Although not a true source of reimbursement per se, this funding had the practical effect of subsidizing operations. As third party reimbursement began to proliferate, the cumulative effect was to reduce the incentive to plan for capital to maintain and acquire assets.

Especially harmful was the notion that costs could be subsidized by third parties. Capital costs were passed to third parties directly due to liberal reimbursement policies. The net result was higher health care costs because no controls were present to hold down either operating or capital costs. Capital asset management therefore became divorced from sound operations management. Gradually the rising cost of hospital construction brought a clearer perspective. Hospitals came to realize that fiscal solvency was related not only to expanding plant and equipment but also to solid management of those assets.

The introduction of health planning and the limitations on Hill-Burton funding contributed to further caution in fiscal management and capital asset planning. Health planning (via certificate of need legislation) prevented unabridged construction in the health field, although its actual impact has been questioned. Nonetheless it did slow down construction (unfortunately at the same time raising construction costs) and prepared health care executives for the increased regulation soon to follow.

Yet for many hospitals the management response to regulation did not come soon enough. Health policy was gravitating rapidly toward control over reimbursement. Major third party payers were no longer accepting a cost-pass-through situation. Growing restrictions motivated more cost shifting among patients and the proliferation of creative accounting.

The culmination of these events and trends was the passage of prospective payment legislation. Although not universally adopted throughout the United States, the prospective payment principle is the basis behind most third party payment plans and is likely to spread to others in the future. The implications for total financial operations are extensive, but they can be reduced to basically two concepts: (1) cost containment and (2) return on investment. It is in this context that a new approach to capital budgeting must be forged. For nurse administrators this is a challenging situation. They must learn traditional capital budgeting and financial management practices, but they must also be prepared to adapt these concepts to the future. Learning the basics of capital budgeting (or any other financial management concept) is only the beginning. Those ideas must be integrated with other financing ideas and then tempered in view of the health care environment.

EROSION OF HOSPITAL CAPITAL

If capital budgeting plans must be created in light of the external environment (and remain compatible with internal organizational goals), an understanding of the erosion of the capital base in the hospital industry is crucial. The problem is especially germane to hospitals but has implications for other health care organizations. Basically the problem is this: hospitals have not been maintaining the value of their capital assets. This problem partially stems from underreimbursed depreciation—the expense for deterioration of plant and equipment—on a historical cost basis.[1] These funding mechanisms could not allow hospitals to keep pace with the severe inflation in hospital construction costs.

Many hospitals turned to debt to fund capital investments. The introduction of revenue bonds (particularly tax-exempt revenue bonds) helped many hospitals to fund capital needs, especially for construction of facilities. There was a major problem in this approach: long-term debt is acceptable leverage to maintain a capital position, but only if there is a sound means of covering the debt expenses. The failure to develop a mind-set of strong fiscal responsibility (i.e., avoidance of debt) over the last few decades has sorely jeopardized future operations. Leverage may be a weak strategy for hospitals because:

- Third party payers have restricted the amount of reimbursement they will pay for depreciation and for return on investment, thus making it difficult to cover debt expenses.
- Operationally, hospitals have not been managed from a businesslike perspective. Consequently the state of the art in control and accountability leaves much to be desired. This makes it more difficult to cover debt through current operations.
- Sources of low-cost capital (notably philanthropy and government programs) have decreased in recent years, leaving no easy solutions for hospitals that have reached a critical capital position.
- The trends indicate greater restriction on the revenue side of hospital operations combined with growing competition among providers for inpatients. Hospitals therefore confront new challenges that require resource investments (e.g., market research and advertising) and make debt funding difficult. With less revenue, hospitals have fewer funds to cover the cost of long-term debt.

Given these pressures, it is easy to see that maintaining a strong capital base is difficult. These difficulties eventually filter down into all levels of the organization. Nursing services are often asked to bear a large portion of the consequences even though they may have little to do with the initial causes or mismanagement of strategic response.

The bottom line to these pressures is what Cleverley terms the erosion of hospital capital.[2] According to his estimates, it is not realistic for hospitals either to maintain or expand their capital base under Medicare reimbursement. Like other forecasters, he suggests that hospitals will turn to debt. With long-term debt, the period required for repaying the debt is usually much shorter than the life of the asset. As long as the asset life is relatively long, hospitals could survive by using long-term debt.[3]

Capital Budgeting Options

The magnitude of the capital erosion problem and its implications for realistic capital budgeting are apparent in the following estimates based on 1980 dollars for 5,842 acute care community hospitals:[4]

Undepreciated fixed capital assets in 1966	= $ 68.2 billion
Adjusting historical costs for inflation (to 1980)	= $123.3 billion
Adjusting for higher construction indexes (to 1980)	= $125.7 billion
Adjusting for technological complexity (to 1980)	= $150.4 billion

The adjustments to the hospital capital base result in assets worth more than twice the initial investment. Balanced against this current value is the allowable depreciation permitted by Medicare or Medicaid. On a historical cost basis depreciation would have been reimbursed at a level of *$20.4 billion.*

The problem clearly is significant. Depreciation has accelerated without commensurate adjustment at the funding level. Bradford, Caldwell, and Goldsmith argue that hospitals should annually depreciate assets at 4 percent of the capital base.[5] Using the 1980 estimated value of hospital assets ($150.4 billion), hospitals would have had to set $63.4 billion aside for depreciation. This has not been done. Nor is there any guarantee that reimbursed depreciation was targeted for capital maintenance instead of other operations. The issue distills to one of determining options for capital budgeting. How does a hospital accumulate capital or attain funds to service debt under these conditions?

There are at least three resolutions to these capital budgeting and financing problems:

- *Current Operations.* A logical source of debt service is internal or current operations. Under this approach, health care facilities would pursue greater fiscal responsibility in operations. They would attempt to operate as efficiently as possible and contain all costs in order to (internally) fund investments in *prioritized* capital budgets. This alternative is congruent with traditional business methods and may be feasible where health institutions adopt more austere plans and a more limited scope of service.
- *Corporate Alliances.* There has been tremendous growth in multi-institutional alliances in the health field and in related joint ventures at the corporate level. These alliances are promising in their ability to match available capital with needs. The infusion of capital makes effective capital budgeting more likely because a health facility may have had numerous options prior to the alliance, but no means for pursuing those options. Corporate alliances are taking many different shapes. This variability will confuse the capital budgeting process. However, without the new sources of capital, there would be little or no budgeting at all.
- *Stock Offerings.* The health field is gradually moving toward a corporate profile. In some sectors the transformation of voluntary and nonprofit orientation to publicly held ventures is progressing rapidly. With stock offerings come the potential for a larger capital investment (from sale of stock) and

hence for an expanded capital budget. There is an accompanying market imperative for better adherence to budgets to maintain financial stability and attractiveness to potential investors.

The possible resolutions to the capital financing and capital budgeting problems in the health care fields call for innovative strategies. In view of the constraints, this innovation is necessary to produce a financially balanced position for long-run survival.

Outlook under Prospective Payment

The outlook for capital financing and capital budgeting under prospective payment is uncertain. Medicare's DRG system initially evaded the issue of capital reimbursement (currently these costs are passed through) and as a result caused considerable confusion for capital budgeting within hospitals. It is difficult to formulate a capital budget if the long-term rate of reimbursement is not known. However, most hospitals have been able to overcome this obstacle because the percentage of Medicare patients served is small.

A more significant issue is the effect of Medicare's DRG system on other prospective payment plans. DRGs may not be around forever, but some type of prospective payment—probably capitated—will dominate reimbursement policy in the health field. How will prospective payment address capital reimbursement? Obviously no one knows at this point, and speculation suggests that any one of a dozen alternatives may be adopted.

In all probability health care providers will not wait for reimbursement policy to be finalized before formulating their long-run capital budgets. Health care organizations have more than just regulation or reimbursement to worry about. With growing competition in the health field and diversification into new service areas, health care organizations cannot delay capital budgeting. They must proceed with their capital budgeting plans and adjust them as reimbursement policy is set in the future. This may not be an optimal approach, but it is realistic.

Nurse administrators should be cognizant of these trends and should continue to monitor their development in future years. By remaining alert to new policy developments, nurse administrators will be able to translate capital reimbursement policies into specific implications for their organizations, departments, or programs. They will be better prepared to formulate meaningful budgets and to act as effective advocates for nursing interests. Their input into the capital budgeting process will proceed from a point of information and assessment rather than speculation.

PLANNING CAPITAL BUDGETS

There is a question of whether hospitals and other health care facilities really need to implement techniques such as capital budgeting.[6] The problem involves the goals of health care organizations. As many nurse administrators recognize, those goals are oriented toward serving human health care needs rather than organizational needs for profit and growth. The argument suggests that health care organizations are not driven toward fiscally optimal performance because the conflict between quality of care and profitability results in priority being given to service. Efficiency and profitability are often sacrificed for quality of care. But are they?

The last five years have presented a surprising change of events in the health field that has converted traditional assumptions into a new set of operating principles. In essence the health field is struggling to define the boundaries of a trade-off between cost and quality in order to direct hospital and health care operations. Cost and return on investment are two dominant concepts that are receiving wide support in planning for hospital operations. This does not imply that values among health care executives have necessarily changed, only that various pressures have driven health care organizations toward a more financially oriented perspective. This is largely the result of policy changes by third party payers.

The implications for capital budgeting are numerous. Organizational goals should guide the priority assigned to specific capital investments. This is more than just an academic argument for specifying goals and ranking them. Since health care organizations cannot hope to fund all projects, they must selectively pursue those that help them attain their most important objectives. Yet how can this occur if organizations themselves are uncertain about what their goals really are? In the confusing and often changing balance between quality of care, level of services, cost, and profitability, inevitably some uncertainty will be transferred to the capital budgeting process. Consequently the selection of which capital projects to fund may proceed without a consistent rationale because the organization itself is uncertain about the direction it is heading.

In terms of capital budgeting, this confusion in goal specificity is of particular concern because most capital investments are designed with the long run in mind. A health care organization must be prepared to live with the results of its decisions for a long time. Thus, it should be evident that everything must be done to carefully establish priorities for guiding decisions. Many health care executives are unwilling to undertake this sort of analysis because it appears to accomplish few tangible results. Quite the contrary is true. The give and take of discussions and analysis of organizational goals may require a substantial investment of staff time, but it is effort well spent. Organizations need to know who they are and where they are going. It is too easy to meander along without conscious resolution of these issues. When confronted by exceptionally perverse pressures—such as high competition and the constraints of prospective payment—the organization must be prepared to respond in the best fashion possible.

Planning for capital budgets cannot be successfully completed when there is uncertainty on the future directions of the organization.[7,8] This is easily seen in the data-gathering phase underlying capital budget planning. A typical analytical approach is to first gather data on budget requests from relevant programs, departments, and management members as illustrated in Table 8–1.

When several clinical departments present their own diverse capital requests, it does not take too long to realize that possible expenditures exceed existing funds or funds available through leverage. The capital requests committee (i.e., the chief executive officer, chief financial officer, chairman of the board, board members, and relevant management staff) reviewing these requests should have an overall capital plan. Goals must be specified in advance; otherwise the organization will incrementally determine its expenditures on capital assets. When resources are plentiful, an ad hoc approach works very well. But in an otherwise austere period of prospective payment, long-run investments must proceed with careful attention to debt service.[9]

The fact that the managers proposing the capital equipment and facilities must prioritize their needs can help the committee to select projects to fund. However, the committee must also be cautious to avoid approving an item from each department, program, or reporting unit. Approving at least one capital budget item from each department is not a discriminating selection process.

Table 8–1 does not indicate that department heads and program directors undertake sophisticated analysis of their projects other than in terms of estimating the costs and benefits/revenues from a given investment. The initial request for data exemplified in Table 8–1 is only a first cut in planning the capital budget. It

Table 8–1 Expenditure Requests for Capital Equipment and Facilities

Equipment or Physical Plant Required	Rationale	Estimated Cost	Estimated Revenue	Justification	Priority
1.					
2.					
3.					
4.					

Added Comments for Consideration:

provides the capital budget committee, finance committee, or other responsible authority for decision making with a *first cut* at planning a capital budget. This initial effort should occur very early in the budgeting process—perhaps as early as in the first quarter of the prior budgeting cycle. This initial assessment can then target the feasible investments within the entire range of opportunities. From this point, department heads and program directors can be asked to document fully the requests that the capital budget committee believes may be seriously considered for funding.

Choosing among Proposals

Once presented with a list of capital expenditure proposals and assuming that funds are available for at least one project, the capital budget committee must reach a decision about funding. The use of objective financing criteria is encouraged in choosing among projects. However, to suggest that financial analysis is the ultimate framework for assessing capital expenditures is not realistic. There are, and always will be, subjective criteria that should be acknowledged in any financial assessment. By developing a well-structured approach to the assessment of capital expenditures both subjective and objective criteria can be considered.[10]

Objective Criteria

Usually investment decisions require a selection among several projects whose values are difficult to compare. In other cases a single expenditure request offers several possible paths and options that must be considered. The advantage of using objective criteria in these situations is to reduce ambiguity and to increase the degree of comparability. When objective criteria are employed it may be possible to differentiate between investments in a lithotripter and in a parking structure in specific monetary terms, patients serviced, externalities (i.e., secondary revenues), or other so-called hard measures of assessmesnt. The difficult comparison is made easier because the analysis is couched in comparable units.

Many objective measures can be used in the capital budgeting process to choose among alternative proposals. Typical examples include the payback method, internal rate of return, average rate of return, and present worth method. These methods will be discussed at length, but for the moment it is important to understand that these powerful methods can be supplemented by specifying as many subjective and objective criteria as possible. Whatever the technique, the critical point to remember is that objective assessment can aid decision making. It does not automatically result in better decisions, but it does facilitate the selection among many alternatives.

Subjective Criteria

Although managers should theoretically be using objective criteria in assessing capital expenditure proposals, the truth is that subjective criteria are used in an exceptional number of instances. There is nothing wrong with including these criteria in an assessment. In fact there is everything right with employing subjective criteria as part of an analysis. The problem is that subjective criteria often prevent comparison. They tend to confuse the choice between one proposal and another. The choice between a lithotripter and parking structure mentioned earlier offers a perfect example.

How does the capital budget committee select between a lithotripter and a parking structure? Assume each will cost $2 million and that the financing costs and debt service are essentially equal. At this point more subjective criteria begin to dominate the decision process. Among other subjective criteria, the following factors may be used in the ultimate selection:

- The hospital auxiliary will raise contributions for the parking structure.
- Adverse parking conditions for physicians have caused some of them to terminate staff privileges.
- Long-run plans to construct a new wing might reduce available parking.
- The limited urosurgical practice in the hospital necessitates opening medical staff privileges in order to raise utilization.
- The chief of staff is a urologist.
- The chairman of the board has purchased a new Mercedes.

These and other subjective criteria are relevant to any decision. It is important to acknowledge that these criteria are often held in higher esteem than seemingly irrefutable objective criteria—even financial assessment criteria.

RANKING INVESTMENT PROPOSALS

Other than the subjective and objective criteria mentioned above for ranking investment proposals, several analytical financial methods can be used in the capital budgeting process. However, before the investment ranking methods can be clearly understood, it is essential that nurse administrators have a firm grasp of the time value of money. Since money has a given value for a period of time, this time value must be incorporated in the analysis. There are various methods for computing this, some more accurate than others. However, others are often used more frequently despite their simplicity. The nurse administrator must be familiar with all of these techniques as well as their advantages and disadvantages.

Compound Interest

Compound interest conveys the fact that money is valuable over time at a given rate of interest. For example, assume that a medical clinic borrows $1,000 for a laboratory microscope over a period of three years. The lender charges 14 percent interest on the loan. How much interest is compounded over the three years? The amount can be calculated as follows:

Year	Interest Rate		Compounded Amount		Interest
1	.14	×	$1,000	=	$140.00
2	.14	×	1,140	=	159.60
3	.14	×	1,299.60	=	181.94
					$481.54

As this illustration indicates, the medical clinic must pay $481.54 in annually compounded interest over the term of the loan. The compound factor increases the yearly interest charged by $61.54 over simple interest. If simple yearly interest were charged the interest cost would be $140 × 3 years = $420. Therefore, the longer the clinic maintains this loan, the higher will be its compounded interest. In the final analysis the microscope actually cost $1,481.54 compared with its purchase price of $1,000.

In financial theory, the concept of compound interest is expressed symbolically as:

$$CS = P(1 + i)^n$$

Where: CS = compound sum
P = principal or present amount
i = interest rate for a given time period
n = number of periods

Using the example for the laboratory microscope:

$$CS = \$1,000 (1 + .14)^3$$
$$CS = \$1,000 (1.482)$$
$$CS = \$1,482$$

From a practical standpoint, an abbreviated formula can be used which is expressed as:

$$CS = P(if)$$

Where: CS = compound sum
P = principal or present amount
if = interest factor

Tables of factors have already been computed for a given interest rate. This rate is matched with a given number of years at which the interest is compounded. This is

Table 8-2 Compound Sum of $1

Year	1%	2%	3%	4%	5%	6%	7%	8%	9%	10%	11%	12%	13%	14%	15%
1	1.010	1.020	1.030	1.040	1.050	1.060	1.070	1.080	1.090	1.100	1.110	1.120	1.130	1.140	1.150
2	1.020	1.040	1.061	1.082	1.102	1.124	1.145	1.166	1.188	1.210	1.232	1.254	1.277	1.300	1.323
3	1.030	1.061	1.093	1.125	1.158	1.191	1.225	1.260	1.295	1.331	1.368	1.405	1.443	1.482	1.521
4	1.041	1.082	1.126	1.170	1.216	1.262	1.311	1.360	1.412	1.464	1.518	1.574	1.631	1.689	1.750
5	1.051	1.104	1.159	1.217	1.276	1.338	1.403	1.469	1.539	1.611	1.685	1.762	1.842	1.925	2.011
6	1.062	1.126	1.194	1.265	1.340	1.419	1.501	1.587	1.677	1.772	1.870	1.974	2.082	2.195	2.313
7	1.072	1.149	1.230	1.316	1.407	1.504	1.606	1.714	1.828	1.949	2.076	2.211	2.353	2.502	2.660
8	1.083	1.172	1.267	1.369	1.477	1.594	1.718	1.851	1.993	2.144	2.305	2.476	2.658	2.853	3.059
9	1.094	1.195	1.305	1.429	1.551	1.689	1.839	1.999	2.172	2.358	2.558	2.773	3.004	3.252	3.518
10	1.105	1.219	1.344	1.480	1.629	1.791	1.967	2.159	2.367	2.594	2.839	3.106	3.395	3.707	4.046
11	1.116	1.243	1.384	1.599	1.710	1.898	2.105	2.332	2.580	2.853	3.152	3.479	3.836	4.226	4.652
12	1.127	1.268	1.426	1.601	1.796	2.012	2.252	2.518	2.893	3.138	3.499	3.896	4.335	4.818	5.350
13	1.138	1.294	1.469	1.665	1.886	2.133	2.410	2.720	3.066	3.452	3.883	4.363	4.898	5.492	6.153
14	1.149	1.319	1.513	1.732	1.980	2.261	2.579	2.937	3.342	3.797	4.310	4.887	5.535	6.261	7.076
15	1.161	1.346	1.558	1.801	2.079	2.397	2.759	3.172	3.642	4.177	4.785	5.474	6.254	7.138	8.137
20	1.220	1.486	1.806	2.191	2.653	3.207	3.870	4.661	5.604	6.728	8.062	9.646	11.523	13.744	16.36
25	1.282	1.641	2.094	2.666	3.386	4.292	5.429	6.849	8.623	10.835	13.586	17.000	21.231	26.462	32.91
30	1.348	1.811	2.427	3.243	4.322	5.744	7.612	10.063	13.268	17.449	22.892	29.960	39.116	50.950	66.21

presented in Table 8–2. Remaining with the laboratory microscope illustration, read across the top of Table 8–2 to locate the interest rate (i.e., 14%). Read down the column to locate the number of years (i.e., 3). The interest factor is .482, which then must be added to 1.00 (to account for the total principal).

A variation on the compounding of interest is to determine how long it takes to double a given principal at a given interest rate. In other words, if $10,000 is invested at 9 percent, how long will it take before the principal is doubled? A convenient decision rule is the rule of 72. It requires the following steps:

1. Divide 72 by the interest rate.
2. The resultant figure is the number of years required to double a given amount.

In the case of $10,000 invested at 9 percent, it is apparent that it will require eight years to double that amount if it is invested at the given interest rate. Remember this is just a convenient decision rule. There are more precise methods for accurately determining the number of years required to double a sum of money.[11]

Present Value

The reverse of a compounded sum is known as the present value (or present worth). Instead of calculating an ending compound sum ($1,481.54 for the laboratory microscope), the initial principal is determined. It is necessary only to revise the formula for the compound sum:

$$P = \frac{CS}{(1 + i)^n} \quad \text{or} \quad P = CS \frac{1}{(1 + i)^n}$$

Where: P = principal or present amount
CS = compound sum
i = interest rate for a given period of time
n = number of periods

In the example of the laboratory microscope we know that it will cost $1,481.54 to purchase the microscope at the end of three years at 14 percent interest, but we wish to know what initial principal must be borrowed. It is calculated in the following fashion:

$$P = 1,482 \frac{1}{(1 + .14)^3}$$
$$P = 1,482 (.675)$$
$$P = \$1,000$$

Once again, tables of factors have been developed for the present value factors. Table 8–3 presents the present values of $1 for associated interest rates and time periods.

Table 8–3 Present Value of $1

Year	1%	2%	3%	4%	5%	6%	7%	8%	9%	10%	11%	12%	13%	14%	15%
1	.990	.980	.971	.962	.952	.943	.935	.926	.917	.909	.901	.893	.885	.877	.870
2	.980	.961	.943	.925	.907	.890	.873	.857	.842	.826	.812	.797	.783	.769	.756
3	.971	.942	.915	.889	.864	.840	.816	.794	.772	.751	.731	.712	.693	.675	.658
4	.961	.924	.889	.855	.823	.792	.763	.735	.708	.683	.659	.636	.613	.592	.572
5	.951	.906	.863	.822	.784	.747	.713	.681	.650	.621	.594	.567	.543	.519	.497
6	.942	.888	.838	.790	.746	.705	.666	.630	.596	.564	.535	.502	.480	.456	.432
7	.933	.871	.813	.760	.711	.665	.623	.583	.547	.513	.482	.452	.425	.400	.376
8	.923	.853	.789	.731	.677	.627	.582	.540	.502	.467	.434	.404	.376	.351	.327
9	.914	.837	.766	.703	.645	.592	.547	.500	.460	.424	.391	.361	.333	.308	.284
10	.905	.820	.744	.676	.614	.558	.508	.463	.422	.386	.352	.322	.295	.270	.247
11	.896	.804	.722	.650	.585	.527	.475	.429	.388	.350	.317	.287	.261	.237	.215
12	.887	.788	.701	.625	.557	.497	.444	.397	.356	.319	.286	.257	.231	.208	.187
13	.879	.773	.681	.601	.530	.469	.415	.368	.326	.290	.258	.229	.204	.182	.163
14	.870	.758	.661	.577	.505	.442	.388	.340	.299	.263	.232	.205	.181	.160	.141
15	.861	.743	.642	.555	.481	.417	.362	.315	.275	.239	.209	.183	.160	.140	.123
20	.820	.673	.554	.456	.377	.319	.258	.215	.178	.149	.124	.104	.087	.073	.061
25	.780	.610	.478	.375	.295	.233	.184	.146	.116	.092	.074	.059	.047	.038	.030
30	.742	.552	.412	.308	.231	.174	.131	.099	.075	.057	.044	.033	.026	.020	.015

Annuities

A more prevalent use of present values and discounting occurs where annuities are involved. An annuity is simply a periodic payment. Periods of payment may be monthly, semiannually, or annually. Using the laboratory microscope example, assume that the equipment produces savings of $600 each year because tissue samples do not have to be sent outside to a contractual agency for analysis. What is the present value of the money that would be saved over the first three years of the microscope?

$$pv = ar \left[\frac{1 - \frac{1}{(1 + i)^n}}{i} \right]$$

Where: pv = present value of the annuity
ar = annual rent or payment
i = interest rate for a given period of time
n = number of years

Using the laboratory microscope example:

$$pv = 600 \left[\frac{1 - \frac{1}{(1 + .14)^3}}{.14} \right]$$

pv = $600 (2.32)
pv = $1,392

The microscope has a present value of $1,392. Another way of calculating this figure is as follows:

Year	Annuity		Present Value Factor		Yearly Savings
1	$600	×	.877	=	$ 526.20
2	600	×	.769	=	461.40
3	600	×	.675	=	405.00
				Total	$1,392.60

Annuity tables have been calculated to prevent excessive effort in determining the value of an annuity received at the end of several years of payment. Table 8–4 presents the present value of an annuity (of $1) received for various years at given interest rates.

The steps to use Table 8–4 are identical to those for the compound sum and present value tables (Tables 8–2 and 8–3 respectively). Ascertain the interest rate on the top row (e.g., 14%) and then determine the period over which the annuity will be received (e.g., 3 years). The factor (i.e., 2.32) is multiplied by the annuity (e.g., $600) to determine the present value or worth of that annuity.

Table 8-4 Present Value of an Annuity of $1

Year	1%	2%	3%	4%	5%	6%	7%	8%	9%	10%	11%	12%	13%	14%	15%
1	0.990	0.980	0.971	0.962	0.952	0.943	0.935	0.926	0.917	0.909	0.901	0.893	0.885	0.877	0.870
2	1.970	1.942	1.913	1.886	1.859	1.833	1.808	1.783	1.759	1.736	1.690	1.713	1.668	1.647	1.626
3	2.941	2.884	2.839	2.775	2.723	2.673	2.624	2.577	2.531	2.487	2.444	2.402	2.361	2.322	2.283
4	3.902	3.808	3.717	3.630	3.546	3.465	3.387	3.312	3.240	3.170	3.102	3.037	2.975	2.914	2.855
5	4.853	4.713	4.580	4.452	4.329	4.212	4.100	3.993	3.890	3.791	3.696	3.605	3.517	3.433	3.352
6	5.795	5.601	5.417	5.242	5.076	4.917	4.766	4.623	4.489	4.355	4.231	4.111	3.998	3.889	3.785
7	6.728	6.472	6.230	6.002	5.786	5.582	5.389	5.206	5.033	4.868	4.564	4.712	4.423	4.288	4.160
8	7.652	7.325	7.020	6.733	6.463	6.210	5.971	5.747	5.535	5.335	5.146	4.968	4.799	4.639	4.487
9	8.566	8.162	7.782	7.435	7.108	6.802	6.515	6.247	5.985	5.759	5.328	5.537	5.132	4.946	4.772
10	9.471	8.983	8.530	8.111	7.722	7.360	7.024	6.710	6.418	6.145	5.889	5.650	5.426	5.216	5.019
11	10.368	9.787	9.253	8.760	8.306	7.887	7.499	7.139	6.805	6.495	6.207	5.988	5.687	5.453	5.234
12	11.255	10.575	9.954	9.385	8.863	8.384	7.943	7.536	7.161	6.814	6.492	6.194	5.918	5.660	5.421
13	12.134	11.348	10.635	9.986	9.394	8.853	8.358	7.904	7.487	7.103	6.750	6.424	6.122	5.842	5.583
14	13.004	12.106	11.296	10.563	9.899	9.295	8.745	8.244	7.786	7.367	6.982	6.628	6.303	6.002	5.725
15	13.865	12.849	11.938	11.118	10.380	9.712	9.108	8.559	8.060	7.606	7.191	6.811	6.462	6.142	5.847
20	18.046	16.351	14.877	13.590	12.462	11.470	10.594	9.818	9.128	8.514	7.963	7.429	7.025	6.623	6.259
25	22.023	19.523	17.413	15.622	14.094	12.783	11.654	10.675	9.823	9.077	8.422	7.843	7.330	6.873	6.464
30	25.808	22.397	19.600	17.292	15.373	13.764	12.409	11.258	10.274	9.427	8.694	8.055	7.496	7.003	6.566

One question that has not been answered in the preceding example of the laboratory microscope is whether the medical clinic should invest in the microscope or not. Under the previously defined conditions, the assessment of the microscope shapes up in this fashion:

Total cost of microscope over 3 years	= $1,482
Present value of savings of microscope over 3 years	= $1,392
Present cost of microscope	= $1,000

If the medical clinic had $1,000 it could immediately invest in the microscope, this would be equivalent to an initial amount of $1,392 or a $392 gain. However, assuming that the clinic must borrow the $1,000, it incurs the interest expense ($482 over three years). From another perspective, by adding the time value of money to the possible yearly savings it is possible to calculate the compounded sum of total savings of the microscope over 3 years:

Year	Interest Rate	Previous Principal + Amount at End of Year		Compounded Amount
1	14%	× $ 600 (accumulated at end of year)	=	$ 600
2	14%	× $ 600 + 600	=	1,284
3	14%	× $1,284 + 600	=	2,063

It is possible to view the $600 annuity as an investment itself if the clinic can take those savings *at the end of each year* and invest them at 14 percent interest. This is a critical assumption because most operating savings are reinvested in operations rather than in new capital assets or marketable investments. There is no interest gained in the first year because it takes the full year to accumulate $600. But this savings can be invested at the beginning of the second year at 14 percent. At the end of the second year, the investment of *savings* has resulted in a compound sum of $1,284. The end of the third year indicates a sum of $2,063. This accumulated or total savings must be compared with the initial investment of $1,000.

Should the clinic invest in the microscope? Given the preceding analysis it is clear that the answer must be in the affirmative. The present value of savings ($1,392) and the total value of savings ($2,063) are favorable when compared with the total cost of the microscope if financed at 14 percent over three years ($1,482). Remember that this analysis has not adjusted for many other factors (criteria) that are relevant to an assessment. Such factors include both subjective and objective criteria:

- Income tax considerations
- Salvage value and depreciable life

- Costs associated with sending laboratory samples out of the clinic to a contracting laboratory
- Time required to wait for test results
- Plans for expansion of clinic use (i.e., higher demand for microscopic examination of samples)
- Staff competency in using the equipment

These and other subjective or objective criteria must be carefully weighed before reaching a final decision on the microscope.

Payback Method

A prevalent method for ranking investment opportunities is to determine how many years are required to return the original investment. The analysis usually incorporates savings before depreciation and after taxes. Although the payback analysis is better than subjectivity or no criteria, it has many weaknesses, including:

- Failure to account for the time value of money
- Inability to recognize that technological obsolescence will render a piece of equipment nonproductive before it reaches its full life
- Predisposition to overlook the efficiency of the equipment in attaining the savings
- Disregard for impact on quality of care

These and other criticisms suggest that the payback method is most useful in estimates of investment attractiveness, but not in a rigorous evaluation of investment opportunities.

Consider the radiology department, which is trying to assess two possible mobile x-ray machines. Assume the following:

1.	*Equipment Model*	*Life*
	Easy Scanner	5 years
	Super Lite	7 years
2.	Cost of capital for the hospital = 10%	
3.	Equipment cost = $10,000 for each model	

The problem is to determine the number of years required to pay back the original investment.

If the machines return the following savings before depreciation, it is possible to calculate their respective payback periods:

Year	Savings Before Depreciation Easy Scanner	Super Lite
1	$5,000	$1,000
2	4,000	2,000
3	3,000	3,000
4	1,000	4,000
5	500	5,000
6		5,000
7		5,000
Payback:	3 years	4 years

The criterion is the number of years required to return the original investment of $10,000. The Easy Scanner requires three years ($5,000 + $4,000 + $3,000) whereas the super Lite takes four years ($1,000 + $2,000 + $3,000 + $4,000) to return the investment. The radiology department should purchase the Easy Scanner.

A problem with the payback method is evident in the number of years of earning capacity that come after payback of initial principal has been made. The Super Lite continues to return substantial savings for three years after the Easy Scanner. This difference is attributable perhaps to a technological characteristic as well as the learning required by the radiology staff. This factor—a valuable consideration—is left out of the analysis. On the other hand, it must be remembered that radiology equipment can become obsolete very rapidly. Therefore the Easy Scanner is somewhat undervalued in the payback analysis. The Super Lite requires an extraordinary amount of time to achieve savings.

Average Rate of Return

Another investment strategy is to calculate the average rate of return. This assessment method is usually defined as:

$$\frac{\text{Sum of Earnings (After Depreciation)}}{\text{Number of Years of Economic Life}} \div \text{Average Investment for the Period} = \text{Average Rate of Return}$$

According to this equation, the return from the investment in a capital asset is adjusted by its economic life and the actual expenditures during the life of the asset.[12,13] For the radiology equipment, the following figures can be used:

Easy Scanner			Super Lite		
Earnings	Depreciation	Earnings After Depreciation	Earnings	Depreciation	Earnings After Depreciation
$5,000	$2,000	$3,000	$1,000	$1,429	$ (429)
4,000	2,000	2,000	2,000	1,429	571
3,000	2,000	1,000	3,000	1,429	1,571
1,000	2,000	(1,000)	4,000	1,429	2,571
500	2,000	(1,500)	5,000	1,429	3,571
		$3,500	5,000	1,429	3,571
			5,000	1,429	3,571
					$14,997

$$\text{Average Rate} = \frac{\$3,500}{5} \div \$5,000 = .14 \qquad \text{Average Rate} = \frac{\$14,997}{7} \div \$5,000 = .43$$

In this comparison between the Easy Scanner and the Super Lite several important assumptions have been made:

- Straight line depreciation is used (five years for the Easy Scanner and seven years for the Super Lite).
- The average investment for the period of use is $5,000 = [($10,000 initial investment + $0 investment at the end of use) ÷ 2]

With this analysis the average rate of return for the Super Lite (43 percent) is over three times that for the Easy Scanner (14 percent). Under these conditions the radiology department should purchase the Super Lite due to its higher rate of return. However, it is important to remember that there are other factors—both objective and subjective—that preclude a simple conclusion on the basis of applying the average rate of return.

Internal Rate of Return

A third investment ranking methodology more powerful than either the payback method or the average return on investment is the internal rate of return. This technique incorporates the time value of money in the assessment of the alternatives. Basically this method requires the calculation of the present value or present worth of a capital asset. The focus is on the interest rate or return generated by the investment—the rate that equates the present value of future returns from the initial investment. In calculating this rate, the nurse administrator will have to experiment with calculations at several interest levels. The criterion again is the interest rate. The higher the interest rate, the higher the internal rate of return. Consequently the better investment has the higher interest rate.

	15% Interest				
Year	*Present Value Factor* *from Table 8–3*	*Easy Scanner*		*Super Lite*	
1	.870	× $5,000 =	4,350	× $1,000 = $	870
2	.756	× 4,000 =	3,024	× 2,000 =	1,512
3	.658	× 3,000 =	1,974	× 3,000 =	1,974
4	.572	× 1,000 =	572	× 4,000 =	2,288
5	.497	× 500 =	249	× 5,000 =	2,485
6	.432		$10,169	× 5,000 =	2,160
7	.376			× 5,000 =	1,880
					$13,169

	22.5% Interest				
Year	*Present Value Factor* *From Table 8–3*	*Easy Scanner*		*Super Lite*	
1	.817	× $5,000 =	$4,085	× $1,000 = $	817
2	.667	× 4,000 =	2,668	× 2,000 =	1,334
3	.546	× 3,000 =	1,638	× 3,000 =	1,637
4	.446	× 1,000 =	446	× 4,000 =	1,784
5	.365	× 500 =	182	× 5,000 =	1,825
6	.299		$9,019	× 5,000 =	1,493
7	.245			× 5,000 =	1,223
					$10,113

Under the two interest rates shown above, the Easy Scanner provides an internal rate of return of approximately 15 percent while the Super Lite provides an internal rate of return of approximately 22.5 percent. Since 22.5 percent is higher than 15 percent, the radiology department should choose the Super Lite as its investment.

The nurse administrator may wonder how the present value factors were ascertained for a 22.5 percent discount rate. Table 8–3 provides information only on 20 and 25 percent. The factors were calculated through interpolation.

Present Worth

A final investment ranking methodology that is useful for nurse administrators to understand is present worth or net present value method.[14] Basically the present worth method determines the present value of all returns from the investment discounted at the cost of capital for the organization. In the radiology department example it was determined that the cost of capital was ten percent. The calculation of present worth proceeds with the idea that this is the rate at which the organization will be charged for capital. Investment of capital should be related to the cost of capital—future earnings are defined in terms of the present value of the organization's capital.

		10% Cost of Capital		
Year	Interest Factor	Easy Scanner	Super Lite	
1	.909	× $5,000 = $ 4,545	× $1,000 = $ 909	
2	.826	× 4,000 = 3,304	× 2,000 = 1,652	
3	.751	× 3,000 = 2,253	× 3,000 = 2,253	
4	.683	× 1,000 = 683	× 4,000 = 2,732	
5	.621	× 500 = 311	× 5,000 = 3,105	
6	.564	Present Worth = $11,096	× 5,000 = 2,820	
7	.513		× 5,000 = 2,565	
			Present Worth = $16,036	

The present worth of the Easy Scanner is $11,096 while the present worth of the Super Lite is $16,036. The decision for investment should clearly be given to the Super Lite due to its high return compared with the radiology department's cost of capital. Per dollar of investment in the Easy Scanner, the radiology department receives a return of 111 percent (i.e., $11,096 ÷ $10,000). Per dollar of investment in the Super Lite, the equipment returns 160 percent (i.e., $16,036 ÷ $11,096). The present value of the Easy Scanner ($11) is less than the present value of the Super Lite ($16). The per dollar investment figure is calculated by dividing the present worth for each asset by the original investment. In the case of the Easy Scanner, the initial dollar investment was $10,000. This investment returned $11,096 or 111 percent ($11,096 ÷ $10,000) of the original investment.

Overview of Investment Ranking

The preceding examples have hinted at the strengths and weaknesses of the investment ranking methods. In the case of the present worth and internal rate of return methods, the time value of money is explicitly incorporated in the analysis. The present worth method directly considers the rate of an organization's cost of capital. For these reasons they must be seen as more legitimate ranking systems. But a judicious analyst should assess major capital investments by as many methods as possible to gain the greatest amount of information on the actual attractiveness of an investment opportunity.

Consider the payback method. Of the four investment ranking procedures, only the payback method recommended investing in the Easy Scanner. All of the other procedures recommended the Super Lite. The lesson to be learned here is that many different dimensions should be assessed—none is the best. Clearly some of the methodologies are more powerful quantitative tools, but that does not mean that they are comprehensive in their analysis. Nurse administrators are cautioned to remember this fact and to seek full assessment of capital investments. Do not overanalyze, but also remember to capture all aspects of an investment opportunity consistent with the magnitude of the investments.

Applications in Health Care

To what extent are these financial techniques actually used in the health care industry? Do health facilities actually evaluate capital investments through either the payback, average rate of return, internal rate of return, or present worth methods? Or is an entirely different set of criteria used? There has been relatively little research in this area, but some evidence is available. It is appropriate to examine these data and gain an appreciation of where health care organizations are in their capital budgeting efforts.

Williams and Rakich sent questionnaires on investment evaluation practices to controllers in 801 short-stay hospitals in 1973.[15] Since this study is dated, caution must be used in interpreting the data. But these data do establish a baseline of sorts. The study attained a 31.6 percent response rate—253 usable responses—which further limits confidence in the results. The data indicate the following ranking of evaluation techniques from the approach most often to least often used:

1. Payback (48.2 percent)
2. Other (33.9 percent)
3. Average rate of return (15.8 percent)
4. Net present value (8.3 percent)
5. Internal rate of return (3.2 percent)

Note that some of the respondents indicated that several techniques were used in their hospitals.

The data provide a rather disappointing profile on the use of rigorous evaluation methods for capital budgeting. The payback method is the most widely used technique despite its many inherent limitations. Almost half of the hospitals use this method. The more sophisticated techniques—especially net present worth and internal rate of return—are hardly used at all. This is very discouraging from the perspective of good management practice.

The intriguing aspect of these data is the "other" category. Over one-third of the controllers indicate that they use some evaluation method other than those listed. What these other techniques consist of is open to speculation. Considering the failure to indicate the use of more sophisticated methods, it may be that the hospitals use other techniques that are less sophisticated. Some examples include:

• Jury of executive opinion—committee decisions
• Cost analysis
• Availability of funds
• No analysis whatsoever

The point is that there is no way of really knowing what "other" implies, but it is most likely that the so-called "other" techniques were probably not rigorous analytical techniques.

Williams and Rakich further analyzed the data to ascertain whether the type of hospital—nongovernmental or governmental, profit or nonprofit—had any influence on the evaluation techniques used. They concluded that there were no consistent, significant differences. In fact they imply that the state of the art in the use of evaluation approaches within hospitals is rather rudimentary. These results and conclusions are fairly well replicated in a study of Ohio hospitals by Williams in 1974.[16,17] Thus, over a decade ago it was apparent that hospital controllers did not envision their organizations as being very rigorous in the application of evaluation methodologies. The question is why?

In the mid–1970s there was less incentive to control expenditures than there is today. In fact Medicare and Medicaid funding was probably very influential in shaping the evaluation techniques used (or not used) at that time. This flush funding environment is undoubtedly responsible for the relatively limited use of sophisticated investment evaluation methods. Would we expect to find similar results today if we replicated the Williams and Rakich studies? The answer is no.[18–20] Hospitals have more pressure to make wise purchase decisions. Prospective payment and other reimbursement changes are influencing financial operations as never before. Whether this pressure has led to greater sophistication in evaluation of capital investments, however, remains to be demonstrated in research. From a practical perspective, hospitals vitally need to apply these techniques if they expect to make good decisions—whether competitors are performing similarly or not.

SUBSTITUTING LEASING FOR CAPITAL EXPENDITURES

Instead of purchasing capital assets, health care organizations can lease them. This is true from the smallest piece of equipment to the largest medical center—all of these assets can be leased just as well as they can be purchased. In order for nurse administrators to know when it is better to lease than to buy, it is essential to know about the various types of leases and why health care organizations are choosing them. The nurse administrator must also be familiar with the conditions under which a lease is reimbursable. This is a highly significant fact that differentiates health care capital budgeting from other business operations—discretion must be used to maximize reimbursement of capital assets.

Types of Leases

A lease differs from a purchase in that ownership is not transferred between parties. The lessor (owner of the asset) transfers to the lessee the rights to use the asset. In return for these rights, the lessee is obliged to make certain payments, often of a periodic nature. There are many different types of leases, many of which ultimately resemble purchases or actually transfer ownership after a given period of leasing.

Operating Lease

The operating lease is typically a contract written for an asset where the lessor provides services relating to the asset. In the health field radiology, diagnostic, and treatment equipment can be obtained through leases. The lessor may provide maintenance, tax coverage, or other services during the lease period. An operating lease is generally for a short time period that is less than the life of the asset. This feature is especially valuable for medical equipment that has a tendency for technological obsolescence. The health care organization can continually retain the latest equipment, albeit at a higher cost than purchasing. Finally, the operating lease is generally more flexible on terms of cancellation.

Financial Lease

A financial or capital lease is an agreement between the lessor and lessee for extended use of an asset. As a result, the lease is often fully amortized in terms of the original purchase price of the asset. Since a financial lease is mainly designed to provide access to the asset, rather than support the maintenance of the asset, there is usually no covenant for a service agreement. However, service or maintenance contracts are often negotiated as part of the lease itself.

A distinguishing characteristic of the financial lease is a renewal option at the end of the lease term. The lessee may have the option to renew the lease. In many instances the lessee is also provided the option to purchase the asset at the termination of the lease. In this manner the lessee is able to retain use of the equipment. This may be highly significant to a health care facility that has altered the physical configuration of its structure in order to use the asset (e.g., a computerized axial tomographic scanner).

These added rights of the lessee are accompanied by added responsibilities. Like debt financing, failure to make lease payments can result in litigation. The lessor will pursue damages for failure to fulfill the term of the lease and will likely retrieve the asset itself. The financial lease therefore is more like purchasing an asset. It involves a greater risk because a contractual agreement is established for a specific period of time.

Sale-and-Leaseback

Under a sale-and-leaseback arrangement, a health care organization will sell an asset to another party (such as a financial institution) and then lease the asset back.

This lease arrangement serves as a quasi-substitute for debt financing. On one hand the lessee has arranged for continued access to the equipment, but on the other hand the lessee has not tied up substantial amounts of liquid assets in the asset. The leaseback will result in a higher premium than if the lessee just retained the asset after purchase because the lessor adds a fair rent to the lease agreement. In many instances the sale-and-leaseback contains a provision for repurchase of the asset by the lessee at the end of the term of the lease. Hence the health care organization can retain both possession and ownership of sorts.

Motivation for Leasing

The large number of types of leases suggests something about the increasing interest by health care organizations in this method of procuring plant and equipment. Nurse administrators need to understand the motivation underlying the adoption of leasing contracts in order to more fully appreciate the financial potential of leasing. Among other factors, health care leasing has grown to such proportions because of the following:[21,22]

- Reimbursement coverage. Under certain conditions the costs of hospital leases are reimbursable by third parties. Reimbursement minimizes the differences between leased assets and purchased assets. Until leases were reimbursed, there was greater incentive to purchase assets in order to recover costs from third party payments.

- Improved service. The lease contract provides a built-in incentive for vendors or owners of assets to offer a high level of service. The lessee has the ability to terminate a lease. Since the lessor derives income from the lease there is an incentive to keep the lessee satisfied with the leased asset.

- Access to capital. Leases provide a convenient source of capital. Without this quasi-source of capital, a health care organization might not otherwise have sufficient capital to purchase an asset. If an organization is able to derive revenues to cover the operating cost (i.e., cost of lease plus associated costs), it may also have an opportunity to attain net profits. These profits would not be available unless the asset were available. Consequently, the lease is an immediate source of capital.

- Management of technological obsolescence. Leases allow health care organizations to turn over equipment much more rapidly than if equipment (or facilities) were purchased. The term of the lease can be managed by the lessee, thereby limiting its commitment to a given piece of equipment. Since medical care technology is rapidly being improved, leasing gives a health care organization early access to the latest technological developments.

Formerly organizations purchasing plant or equipment had to be more conservative in the turnover of these assets in order to break even on the purchases.

- Lower discount rates. Leases are sometimes lower in cost as far as interest rates are concerned. When interest rates are very high for borrowing money, many lessors are able to be very competitive in the added costs for interest in their lease charges. However, when interest rates decline, the reverse occurs and leasing tends to be more costly than outright purchasing as far as interest rates are concerned.

Leasing, therefore, provides several incentives to health care facilities to acquire assets that may not otherwise be obtainable. Nurse administrators must recognize that leasing is not necessarily better than purchasing assets, or vice versa. Rather, a comprehensive view of the financial solvency of an organization must be considered in relation to the purpose and demand for the asset and the ability to improve overall profitability. In some situations other strategic criteria should be integrated in the leasing decision. Market competitiveness is a perfect example of these additional criteria.

Is a Lease Reimbursable?

Nurse administrators should be alert to whether a lease is reimbursable from third parties. It should not be assumed that any given lease will necessarily be covered by third party payments. Before entering into the lease, some investigation is appropriate. At issue here are revisions in standards by the Financial Accounting Standards Board, specifically Standard 13, "Accounting for Leases" (FAS 13). Since third party payers adopt the standards of the Financial Accounting Standards Board, the health care organization as a potential lessee must determine whether the lease will fall into one of two categories:

1. Financial lease. The asset is recorded on the organization's balance sheet as an asset and balanced as a liability in terms of lease payments owed.
2. Operating lease. The asset remains off the balance sheet.

A financial or capital lease will alter the financial profile of the health care organization because it implies higher recorded debt. The operating lease does not affect the financial profile in such a dramatic way. From the third party payer's perspective, the capital lease will result in early payments at an accelerated rate. There are also significant implications for reversing this cash flow advantage in later years due to costs that exceed reimbursement limitations. Nurse administrators must work closely with accountants and third party payers (who will be reimbursing for patient care) to ascertain the precise ruling on lease reimbursement before entering into either a financial or operating lease.

According to Horwitz, the distinguishing features of the financial lease as far as reimbursement are concerned include the following:[23]

- Ownership is transferred to the lessee by the end of the lease term.
- The lease contains a bargain purchase option.
- The lease term is equal to 75 percent or more of the estimated economic life of the lease property.
- The present value at the beginning of the lease term of the minimum lease payment equals or exceeds 90 percent of the excess of any fair value of the leased property over any related investment tax credit obtained by the lessor.

Should *any* of the preceding criteria be met, the lease is treated as a financial lease. This is just the beginning of the reimbursement and accounting implications. Operating leases and financial leases are then differentiated on the basis of depreciation.[24] Operating leases are generally depreciated over the term of the lease, while financial leases are depreciated over the normal life of the asset. Recent changes in generally accepted accounting principals have reduced this disparity.

Financial Impact of Different Leases

The financial impact of operating leases versus financial leases can be readily seen in the balance sheet. Assuming that a hospital has $25 million in plant and equipment, a total debt of $20 million, and revenues of $2.5 million per year, the balance sheet entries would appear as follows where a $3 million lithotripter (with five years' life) is leased under an operating lease:

Balance Sheet for Operating Lease

Assets:	$25,000,000
Debt:	20,000,000
Balance:	$ 5,000,000

The income statement would appear as follows:

Income Statement for Operating Lease

Revenues:	$ 2,500,000
Interest on	
debt—10%	2,000,000
Lease Payment	1,000,000
	($ 500,000)

In the case of the financial lease, the lithotripter would have to be recorded on the organization's books and depreciation added. The balance sheet at year end reflects the addition of both the asset's value and the hospital's increased indebtedness:

	Financial Lease	*Explanation of Adjustment*
Assets:	$27,400,000	Added the asset less straight line depreciation for one year.
Debt:	22,700,000	Debt is amortized by each lease payment (assuming payment of $1 million per year) less any interest = $23,000,000 − ($1,000,000 − 300,000) = $22,700,000.
Balance:	4,700,000	

The income statement would appear as follows:

	Financial Lease	*Explanation of Adjustment*
Revenues	$2,500,000	None
Interest on debt–10%	2,000,000	None
Interest on lease debt at 10%	300,000	Added interest for lease. There is no entry for lease payment.
Depreciation	300,000	Added depreciation.
Balance	($ 100,000)	

The impact on financial ratios is clear:

	Operating Lease		*Financial Lease*	
Return on Assets	$\dfrac{(\$500,000)}{\$25,000,000}$	= −2%	$\dfrac{(\$100,000)}{\$27,400,000}$	= −.36%
Debt to Total Assets	$\dfrac{\$20,000,000}{\$25,000,000}$	= .80	$\dfrac{\$22,700,000}{\$27,400,000}$	= .83

According to these financial ratios, the lithotripter is not a good investment from either the operating lease or financial lease perspective. In the case of the operating lease it does not provide a positive return on assets. In the case of the financial lease it does not provide a positive return on assets and it increases the ratio of debt to total assets. The lithotripter is not a good investment for either lease and it adds greater debt in the case of the financial lease.

Leasing and Nurse Administrators

Nurse administrators will seldom be required to make lease versus purchase decisions on plant or equipment without the assistance of other manageme t staff, consulting accountants, and financial managers. However, this does not diminish the importance of understanding the trade-offs that must be made in acquiring assets. In substituting leasing for capital expenditures, nurse administrators shculd contemplate:

- the type of lease involved
- the relevance and priority of factors that motivate leasing over purchasing
- the extent to which the lease or purchase would be reimbursable from third party payers
- the treatment of the lease by accounting standards and its impact on financial records
- the overall impact on the financial performance of the health care organization

By being cognizant of these factors, the nurse executive is better prepared to contribute to strategic decision making.

SELF STUDY EXERCISES

To improve your skill in capital budgeting, the following exercises are offered to test your command of the ideas presented in Chapter 8. Answers to each question are in Appendix A.

1. A home health agency decided to borrow $20,000 at 12 percent interest payable over five years in order to purchase a marketing study. How much interest was charged over the life of the loan?
2. What is the present value of $2,000 due two years from now, discounted at 7 percent?
3. The nursing department in a large metropolitan hospital decides to immediately terminate ten registered nurses in order to balance the revenue reductions experienced by prospective payment. Assuming that the total yearly salary of these nurses was $287,941 and that the cost of capital for the hospital is 9 percent, what is the present value of the annuity that the hospital saves over a five-year period due to these terminations?
4. A nursing home is contemplating two different models of hydraspas for its patients. The Super Bubbly has a useful life of 3 years while the Quiet

Stream has a longer life of 5 years. The difference in usefulness is due to the types of jet stream and bubbling intensity. The Super Bubbly and the Quiet Stream can each be purchased for $5,000. The cost of capital for the nursing home is 12 percent. The nursing home will charge patients for their use of the hydraspas. The Super Bubbly fills up with water faster and gives a more vigorous treatment in a shorter period of time than the Quiet Stream. Hence, more patients can be treated yearly. Anticipated revenue projections are as follows:

Year	Super Bubbly	Quiet Stream
1	$3,000	$2,000
2	2,500	1,500
3	500	1,500
4		1,500
5		500

Which hydraspa should the nursing home purchase according to the payback and present worth methods of investment ranking?

NOTES

1. R. Neal Gilbert, "Present Value Depreciation: The Answer to the Hospital Capital Crisis?" *Hospital Financial Management* 29 (March 1975): 26–41.
2. William O. Cleverley, "Is Hospital Capital Being Eroded under Cost Reimbursement?" *Hospital Administration* 19 (Summer 1974): 58–73.
3. Wendy M. Greenfield, "Capital Management of the Dilemma of Debt," *Hospital Financial Management* 35 (March 1981): 24–25, 28, 32–33.
4. Charles Bradford, George Caldwell, and Jeff Goldsmith, "The Hospital Capital Crisis: Issues for Trustees," *Harvard Business Review* (September-October 1982): 56–68.
5. William O. Cleverley, "Hospital Capital."
6. Paul L. Bash, "Can Capital Budgeting Work in Hospitals?" *Hospital Administration* 16 (Spring 1971): 59–64.
7. Robert A. Vraciu, "Programming, Budgeting, and Control in Health Care Organizations: The State of the Art," *Health Services Research* 14 (Summer 1979): 126–149.
8. Kenneth Kaufman and Mark Hall, "Strategic Capital Planning, Part II," *Healthcare Financial Management* 37 (April 1983): 97–98.
9. Thomas E. Fitz, "Debt Capacity Analysis is Critical to Planning," *Healthcare Financial Management* 37 (January 1983): 52–58.
10. Kenneth Kaufman and Mark Hall, "Strategic Capital Planning, Part I," *Healthcare Financial Management* 37 (March 1983): 79–80.
11. J.P. Gould and R.L. Weil, "The Rule of 69," *Journal of Business* 49 (July 1974): 397–398.
12. Jonathan W. Pearce, "How To Evaluate the Return on Your Investment," *Healthcare Financial Management* 3 (July 1984): 113–114.
13. Jay Harris and Jim Ruetz, "Rate of Return: A Tool To Evaluate Diversification," *Healthcare Financial Management* 38 (December 1984): 28–34.

14. Jerry Bolandis, "Net Present Value: A Better Way to Evaluate Capital Expenditures," *Hospital Financial Management* 3 (December 1977): 19–28.

15. John D. Williams and Jonathan S. Rakich, "Investment Evaluation in Hospitals," *Financial Management Journal* 2 (Summer 1973): 30–35.

16. John D. Williams, "How Do You Evaluate Capital Investment?" *Hospital Financial Management* 28 (February 1974): 32–35.

17. Carl M. Hubbard, "Capital Budgeting and Cost Reimbursement in Investor-owned and Not-for-Profit Hospitals," *Health Care Management Review* 8 (Summer 1983): 7–17.

18. William O. Cleverley and Joseph G. Felkner, "The Association of Capital Budgeting Techniques with Hospital Financial Performance," *Health Care Management Review* 9 (Summer 1984): 45–58.

19. Alan D. Meyer, "Hospital Capital Budgeting: Fusion of Rationality, Politics, and Ceremony," *Health Care Management Review* 10 (Spring 1985): 17–27.

20. C. Rick Wilson, "The Basics of Budgeting for Capital Equipment," *Hospital Pharmacy* 20 (February 1985): 103–107.

21. James B. Henry and Rodney L. Roenfeldt, "Cost Analysis of Leasing Hospital Equipment," *Inquiry* 15 (March 1978): 33–37.

22. Richard W. Furst, *Financial Management for Health Care Institutions* (Boston, Mass.: Allyn & Bacon, Inc., 1981).

23. Ronald M. Horwitz, "Accounting, Management, Impact of FAS 13: How Will It Affect Paperwork and Reimbursement?" *Hospital Financial Management* 33 (August 1979): 16.

24. Martin E. Zummerman, "Accounting for Lease," *Hospital Financial Management* 33 (June 1979): 26–29.

Chapter 9

Capital Financing

Provisions for capital asset development and financing of new capital projects are serious concerns for any health care organization. Without adequate attention to capital financing it is possible that organizations would lose the capacity to attract clientele due to deteriorating physical plant and equipment. Furthermore, inattention to financing trends can result in higher long-term costs. These factors explain why health care managers must be attentive to capital financing issues.

Nurse administrators can play a significant role in capital financing. They are routinely asked for input on major purchases such as diagnostic and treatment equipment and on facility design. Admittedly, nurse administrators are often omitted from key capital asset decisions such as financing a new hospital building, constructing a clinic, or creating a laboratory. It is not uncommon for chief executive officers themselves to be removed from these issues. Consultants in arranging financing are increasingly being used to produce the financing package for major capital investment by health care organizations. These consultants know the most current trends among funding sources, have access to capital markets, and have experience in arranging the total financing package to the advantage of the organization.

Chief financial officers are typically asked to arrange for *outside* consulting help on financial projects that have significant dollar value. It is not that the chief financial officers lack knowledge about critical financing parameters. The costs attributable to financial staff gaining access to markets and putting together the best financial package are often too high for the organization. It is far preferable to avoid these costs because once a 15-, 20-, or 30-year package is arranged, the health care organization will have to live with the agreement for a long time.

Chief financial officers will often have to arrange financing for expensive capital investments in renovating plant, constructing new additions, or purchasing major pieces of equipment. Financial planning for a $2.5 million magnetic resonance imager can be just as complex as the planning for a $20 million addition to a hospital. The ability to arrange financing is especially needed by financial officers in smaller health care organizations. Their responsibilities are accentuated because the organization usually does not have the resources to procure outside assistance.

Nurse administrators are seldom involved in financial projects to the extent of the chief financial officer or the financial staff. However, this does not mean they can simply overlook capital financing issues. Depending on the size of the health care organization and the level of the nurse administrator in the organizational hierarchy, there may be numerous opportunities to influence capital financing decisions. This opportunity should increase over the next decade as corporate health care organizations evolve.

The nurse administrator in a 250-bed general hospital may have as many opportunities to contribute to financial planning as the chief financial officer or executives in investor-owned corporations. Among the many options for input are the following:

- Advice on the equipment needed in a new facility
- Advice on the redesign of existing facilities that may ultimately influence the cost of a project
- Expert testimony on the trade-offs in function and quality of care from major capital equipment
- Input on the ability of a program, department, or division to raise productivity or lower costs in order to attain net income that can be used for internal financing purposes (e.g., to make loan payments)
- Incorporation of financing issues within a comprehensive approach to managing nursing programs
- Translating the constraints of financing into a forecasted impact on nursing programs—higher costs for financing various projects may culminate in lower operating budgets and greater restraints on raises for personnel
- Recommendations for long-run financial planning as far as the specific capital asset needs of a nursing program, now and in the future

These opportunities are only a few of the many points at which nurse administrators can effectively contribute to the financial planning and decision-making process. Implied within these opportunities is the necessity for nurse administrators to expand their vision of where input can be provided.

SOURCES OF FINANCING

Nurse administrators should be cognizant of the primary sources of financing in order to understand how and why decisions are made about acquiring funding that affect capital assets. It is useful to note that the traditional sources of financing have undergone substantial change in the health care field. From all indications it is probable that changes will continue in the future. As a result, health care organizations can no longer rely on one or two dominant funding sources. Financing increasingly necessitates creative planning. Many factors contribute to the change and uncertainty surrounding capital asset financing.

For years health care facilities relied on philanthropy and government appropriations to fund their capital projects. While philanthropy has gradually decreased as a source of funding, it never was a dominant method for financing projects. There was too much uncertainty surrounding acquisition of funds from this source. Today and in the foreseeable future it appears that many worthy causes (other than just health care) will compete for the charitable contributions of the public. Hence few health care organizations can effectively rely on philanthropy as a main source for funding. Concurrently, the availability of government funding for health care construction has dissipated. There have been increasing pressures on government to curtail costs. The effect has been limits on government investment in health facility construction. Changes in philanthropy and government appropriations have caused hospital and other health care organizations to scramble for financing of major projects.

A temporary substitute for philanthropy and government appropriation was found in the form of tax-free revenue bonds. However, there is serious question how long this alternative will be available. Numerous changes in the tax laws proposed each year could effectively limit the funds available for hospital construction from tax-free revenue bonds. The result is a growing emphasis on corporate financing and use of conventional long-term debt. As we shall see, these trends have profound implications for health care organizations not only in how they are run but also in terms of the type of financial planning that is undertaken.

To hope that revenues will rise to cover debt is a dangerous and perhaps foolish thought. Few indications suggest that third party payers will do anything other than tighten their restrictions on funding. One conclusion seems inevitable— health care organizations will be increasingly forced to finance a portion of capital projects out of current operations. Current operations will be used to service principal and interest payments. Nursing programs will be called on to contribute their fair share to this strategy.

Philanthropy

Donation of private funds for health facility construction has a long and generous history. However, donations have represented only a minor percentage of capital project funding in recent years. This does not imply that philanthropy has diminished in importance, but rather that health care organizations cannot rely on philanthropy from year to year to meet their capital needs. The inability to rely on philanthropy implies that an overall financing strategy must be elucidated. For example, the scale of building costs has escalated to the extent that most philanthropic donors are unable to meet the total financial needs of new construction. As a result, it may be more effective to view these donations as a buffer that facilitates acquisition of a financing package.

According to recent statistics, philanthropy represents approximately 3.9 percent of all sources of financing for hospital construction.[1] Most of this charitable giving is directed toward not-for-profit hospitals, community general hospitals, and nonfederal hospitals. This percentage has been steadily decreasing during the last decade. Such a decline is due partly to the growth of other financing alternatives such as tax-exempt bonds, but the escalating cost of constructing hospitals should also be recognized. For precisely these same reasons, there is ample evidence to believe that philanthropy will decline even further as a source of reliable hospital capital.[2] The impact of inflation is a primary cause for the decrease in importance of philanthropy. At this point the cost of providing a hospital bed has been driven up to the point that health care organizations have to seek funding from sources other than philanthropy.

Government Grants

The hospital industry grew very quickly due primarily to the availability of convenient capital for hospital construction. The Hill-Burton program was important in the effort to expand hospital coverage to communities throughout the United States. These governmental grants and appropriations began to diminish in the early 1970s with the introduction of service-oriented programs such as Medicare and Medicaid, which focused on meeting medical needs of the public rather than on building construction. At the same time health planning was introduced to control the rate of duplicated coverage in many urban areas. Thus, a complex combination of factors forms the present foundation to government capitalization of the health care industry.

Today various government grants account for 12.1 percent of all sources of hospital capital.[3] However, it must be remembered that this figure is inflated as a result of construction of federal hospitals such as in the Veterans Administration. Also included in this percentage is the construction of long-term care hospitals for psychiatric care or for treatment of tuberculosis. It is apparent that governmental sources of funding are not really a viable element in the funding alternatives for hospitals.

This conclusion applies particularly when one considers the many restrictions government grants and appropriations place on health care facilities. It has not been uncommon for the health care organization to be required to pledge ownership of the assets to the government agency at the end of a prespecified term. This loss of ownership is clearly a detrimental aspect of funding through governmental sources. In fact, it is only an unusual case that would motivate a private or nonprofit voluntary hospital to consider such an alternative.

A better appreciation of the extent of government grants and appropriations can be gained by reviewing the prominent past and present sources of financing as follows:[4]

- A state or local public authority issues bonds that are designed to provide funds for specific construction of health care facilities. The funding authority is exempt from federal income tax and in some cases state taxes, which lowers the interest rate for the bond.
- Federal Housing Administration mortgages have been available for health care facility construction. These loans have provided capital when a health care organization does not have extensive capital available for a base. These are situations where lenders would not otherwise be attracted. There are usually stipulations that the facility must provide a particular level of free care.
- The Hill-Burton program offers loan guarantees and subsidization of interest payments. It also offers direct loans. This funding was the basis upon which the present-day hospital industry was built.
- The Government National Mortgage Association, also known as "Ginnie Mae," has been used to sell Federal Housing Administration–backed mortgages to investors. This program is an effort to make mortgages more secure and hence more marketable.
- The Farmers Home Administration has offered some funds to small communities (less than 50,000 population) that need priority public projects.

Although some of these sources are still available, they have generally been reduced in scope and magnitude except for the state or local revenue bonds.

Internal Operations

A prevalent policy in business organizations is to plan for depreciation of plant and equipment and in so doing set aside funds in retained earnings to finance various capital projects. Business corporations do not have the luxury of relying on third party payers to fund the costs of capital. This contribution by third party payers carries with it certain advantages and disadvantages as far as the health care organization is concerned. On one hand health care facilities do not know where their reimbursement of capital asset depreciation will come from because not all third party payers reimburse at the levels needed to compensate for depreciation. On the other hand, reliance on third party payers has created a dysfunctional mind-set in health care management that all costs, including significant capital costs, will be covered by external sources.

A key concept that is missing in the management of health care organizations is autonomy from third party payment. Only prepaid health plans avoid this pitfall.[5] Liberal third party payments that allowed most costs to be reimbursed essentially handed health care executives a blank check. Little control was needed over internal operations or over financial management of capital assets. Costs would eventually be reconciled by reimbursements. Deficits could often be covered by available philanthropy. The profile that emerges is one where health care organizations and their managers experienced little or no incentive to make hard-nosed decisions about cost containment. There was little need to plan for financial needs through efficient operations. Too many easy alternatives existed to cover cost overruns or to acquire capital for maintenance, expansion, or new construction.

For these reasons, health care organizations have overlooked the role of internal operations as a source for funding plant and equipment. This oversight may also be related to the general nonprofit status of the health care industry—there has been little incentive to operate efficiently and little orientation to achieve profitability. As long as this philosophy dominates the management of health care organizations, internal operations will never be placed in their proper perspective.

Internal operations must fund current and future capital investment. This can best be achieved where operations are run with efficiency in mind. Profitability is a prerequisite because it is necessary to cover any future investment and debt on the basis of existing capabilities. Therefore if a hospital wants to invest $20 million in new facilities, it must currently have (or be able to attain in the next fiscal period) surpluses from its operations to cover the costs of capital investment.

This philosophy is vital to nursing administrators. They need to adopt a posture that break-even or zero income performance is insufficient for survival. Health care organizations will increasingly be called upon to run their operations as though they were like any other corporation. In anticipation of this shift, nursing administrators must instill in their staff members the belief that profitable operations are synonymous with survival. Without net income or efficient performance the health care organization will watch its capital position deteriorate.

Such was the case for the United States steel industry, where profits were not reinvested in plant and equipment. Eventually the assets depreciated to the point of obsolescence. Health care organizations not only need to be more highly focused on making profits from internal operations, they also have to be more cognizant of investing these surpluses in plant and equipment. When seen in this light, profitability in the health field is highly critical because profits are a normal part of maintaining the vitality of the organization's assets.

The nonprofit orientation of the health care field with its attendant philanthropy has made it difficult for many organizations to pursue efficient operations. As long as there are subsidies in the form of either philanthropy or government appropriations (e.g., Hill-Burton funds), health care organizations will have difficulty adopting a new outlook that rewards efficiency. To this point, many facilities have been built by nonprofit health care institutions through generous giving. These charitable donations will probably always be part of the health care field. Their intentions and accomplishments are admirable. However, such philanthropy may have inadvertently weakened the ability or desire of some health care managers to work hard in gaining profitable operations.

Some proof of this mind-set of nonprofitability has been presented by Hugh W. Long in his examination of investment decision making by health care organizations.[6] According to Long, private sector health care providers must first consider the cash flows of an investment (e.g., construction of a clinic) and then consider the social good of the investment. Any investment that returns a negative cash flow or net present value should not be funded. This is an excellent point except that it should not be limited solely to for-profit organizations. The current and future health care environment requires *all* organizations to be conscious of, committed to, and actively pursuing profitability in internal operations if they expect to maintain their capital position over the long run.

Nurse administrators could adopt few better ideas than these as a foundation for their financial management practices. Nursing services can make a significant contribution to profits by lowering costs. Surplus income will be increasingly needed to fund investments in plant and equipment. Once those capital assets have been allowed to deteriorate to the point of obsolescence, the health care organization's survival is threatened. It cannot ensure the ability to produce services as it has in the past.

Approximately 15 percent of all hospital construction begun in 1981 was attributable to funds generated from internal operations.[7] These funds represent the total amount of capital invested rather than the percent used to service debt. This is an important distinction for nurse administrators to understand. Assume that a hospital is considering the following investments:

	$15,983,000	new coronary unit
	$ 2,523,000	magnetic resonance imager
	$ 1,617,000	refurbishing existing plant
	$ 108,000	chairs, tables, and cooking equipment for the food service department
	$ 7,894	physical therapy equipment
Total Requests	$20,238,894	

It is possible that if the operations of the hospital were large enough, it could fund all of these projects from its operating surplus. Obviously there are very few hospitals that could fund $20,000,000 in capital assets from one year's performance. Only chains of hospitals could possibly achieve this level of funding. Alternatively, it is possible that a fund could be created for retained earnings to replace plant and equipment. With sufficient efficiency, a hospital could add to this fund each year and thereby achieve a capital asset replacement balance of this magnitude.

These funding mechanisms illustrate the role of internal operations in covering capital asset investment. There is another option as well. Within the list of desirable investments the hospital may decide to use $549,000 of current surplus from operations for investment in the asset base. The decision might allocate $7,894 toward the physical therapy equipment, $108,000 toward the food service investments, and $433,106 toward refurbishing existing plant. Assume that the remaining $19,689,894 of preferred capital investment will be derived from two sources—philanthropy ($1,000,000 fund drive) and long-term debt. The point is that internal operations act as a supplement to capital investment. Without disciplined financial planning and periodic retention of earnings over years of operation, the strategy of using internal operations to fund capital assets will ultimately fail.

Internal operations can also be used to generate payments to cover the principal and interest needed to service long-term debt. But this investment per se is not funding assets through current operations in the sense of periodically saving capital to purchase the assets. In practice, however, this difference may be meaningless. Debt servicing is really just another way of purchasing assets over an extended period of time.

There is an important distinction about which nurse administrators should be aware. To use debt to acquire assets may imply that the organization has not given sufficient forethought to its capital asset needs. Ideally, operations should be managed to retain sufficient earnings to replace assets on a periodic basis. Given the magnitude of most asset acquisition in major facility construction and purchases, this concept is seldom adhered to in practice. Add to this the forces that have stimulated a lax attitude in managing—third party payment, government subsidies, and philanthropy—and it is apparent that most health care organizations will use sources other than internal operations to fund capital asset investment.

Corporate and Multi-Institutional Sources

An increasingly prevalent form of funding for capital assets is through corporate sources. Usually this represents a form of a loan to a health facility that has merged with a corporate chain or a multi-institutional system. As such, these forms of funding really deserve classification as long-term debt. In other cases, venture capital is invested with ownership transfer.[8] Since there is growing activity in the acquisition of capital from multi-institutional and corporate sources, it is appropriate that nurse administrators become familiar with these trends.

A hospital may join a corporate chain for many reasons, one of which is the availability of capital to renovate, expand, or construct new facilities. Part of the merger agreement may stipulate that a given level of capital investment will be made in the hospital's plant and equipment. Consider a nonprofit hospital that is facing a $25 million investment in a new 200-bed facility. Unless it can alter operations to provide sufficient surplus to fund long-term debt, agree to the stipulations covering government appropriations, or successfully mount a significant fund drive, it faces a complex problem. It cannot service debt, yet it faces an environment where reimbursement is requiring more cutbacks and reductions (thereby further jeopardizing ability to service debt over the period of the loan).

An attractive option is to link up with a corporate chain. Most likely, nonprofit status will be sacrificed, but the prospects for covering future debt are unlimited. By joining the corporation the hospital accesses a new pool of capital. This capital may be the result of operating surpluses from the constituents of the corporate chain, it may represent gains from divestment of assets at a profitable level, or there may be funds available from diversification in other business activity. In any case, the hospital has access to a pool of capital not previously available.

Most likely the hospital will have to pay for this capital in the sense of servicing the principal and interest payments. But the cost of this capital will generally be lower than the cost in normal financial markets. This is particularly important if the hospital is in a rural community where its cost of capital will be very high. By joining the chain it may be able to acquire $20,000,000 at New York prime (e.g., 10.25 percent interest) compared with local prime (e.g., 11.75 percent interest). This interest advantage may make the difference in the feasibility of the project.

There are certainly many other significant factors in a decision to join a chain for capital acquisition. Presumably the chain will purchase the assets of the hospital in the merger. As a result the hospital has received a large lump sum for reinvestment. The for-profit chain might pay the historical book value or even market value for the assets—this decision is dependent on the negotiations and goals of both parties. However this transaction occurs, it is apparent that the hospital will be acquiring a large sum of capital. It has given up ownership in return for this capital. Nonetheless, it has derived a means of continuing its operations for the future.

Multi-institutional systems also provide another option for capital that can be used to fund assets. There are many state hospital professional associations that provide access to capital for members. Unlike corporate sources, these funds are usually available only through loans. Thus, they are little more than long-term debt. The point is that involvement of organizational systems in funding capital is growing in the health care field. These opportunities are limited in terms of the capital they provide and also may require a significant abdication of ownership control.

As we have seen, the health care organization is being pressured to switch from operating like a nonprofit organization to a for-profit corporation. There are serious implications for management under such a shift that ultimately will affect daily operations. Nurse administrators are urged to remain alert to the mechanisms by which their organizations acquire capital. They may discover that an eroding asset base has resulted in significant changes in orientation as far as where capital will be acquired in the future.

Long-Term Debt—Taxable

Assuming that a health care organization has decided to use debt to fund its capital assets, it must choose between taxable and nontaxable debt. Under taxable debt, the interest payments received by investors are taxed like other income. Taxation is generally disagreeable to investors. As a result, they may invest their capital in an alternative that provides a good return on investment yet shelters them from a higher tax burden (e.g., treasury notes). In contrast, other investors may be attracted to the rate of return offered through taxable debt and they may prefer the low risk associated with hospital investments. These ideas suggest the present trends in the capital market of the health care field. Capital becomes more available as the rate of return increases and the risk decreases.[9,10]

Because of the imperatives for high rates of return and low risk, fewer hospitals have been using taxable debt to fund operations. In fact, the magnitude of taxable long-term debt used by hospitals has been generally decreasing over the last ten years. The reason for these trends is obvious. Like any other investment situation, hospitals have to compete for capital in the marketplace. Hence capital will be available as long as a sufficient return is offered by low-risk buyers of capital. Suppliers of capital are willing to lend capital as long as their investment criteria of return and risk are met. Since hospitals are generally willing to meet market demands for major equipment purchase, minor construction, renovation, or expansion, there will probably always be moderate involvement in the long-term debt market.

The long-term debt market is flexible and easy to access. It does not carry many of the restrictions that accompany other sources of financing. There are many sellers. For all of these reasons, health care organizations can use the long-term debt market to supplement their overall financial plans. There are other more attractive alternatives for funding major renovation, construction, or expansion of facilities, but these other mechanisms dictate more constraints than health care organizations may be willing to meet. In essence, the taxable long-term debt alternative provides flexibility. With careful shopping at the right moment, this market is quite viable for most health care organizations.

Long-Term Debt—Tax Exempt

The foundation of hospital construction is in tax-exempt revenue bonds, representing over 55 percent of all sources of funds.[11] In comparison, taxable long-term.debt is approximately 14 percent of all funding for hospital construction. The reason hospitals continue to use tax-exempt bonds is their lower cost. Although investors are demanding high interest rates on these bonds, this mechanism still offers two distinct advantages that allow hospitals to pay lower interest rates than for taxable long-term debt. The first advantage is the fact that investors are able to avoid some taxes on their return on investment. The second advantage is that hospitals have offered a relatively risk-free investment. Due to the past stability of third party payments, hospitals were able to offer investors a bond with a high security rating.

Nonprofit community hospitals have been the predominant users of tax-exempt funding. Reliance on tax-exempt funding has been facilitated by legislative activity that permits issuing bonds for the purpose of hospital construction. Changes in the tax laws have gradually made such bonds more attractive to investors. The result is that nonprofit hospitals have come to rely on a single source of funds to assist in capital projects. Whether this strategy will prove to be detrimental to the overall ability of hospitals to maintain their capital position remains to be seen.

There are several trends that threaten hospital financing through tax-exempt bonds. One of the major drawbacks to tax-exempt funding has been its low return to the investor. In periods of inflation the bonds have often caused substantial losses for the holders.[12] The investment community tends to avoid such problems by withholding purchases until the interest rate rises. Consequently it becomes difficult to sell new offerings unless the return is raised—this increases the cost to the hospital and may reduce its ability to meet the obligations. Another drawback to tax-exempt funding is the growing uncertainty over the direction of third party payments. As long as it appears that hospital reimbursement will be restricted in the future, it will be difficult to market tax-exempt bonds. This liability also applies to other forms of long-term debt, but it must be remembered that the tax-exempt bond already must contend with a lower interest rate.

In summary, tax-exempt revenue bonds offer the following features and trends:

- Bonds have become the predominant vehicle for funding hospital construction. Since approximately half of all construction is devoted to renovation of existing plant, the use of this funding is essential to the continued strength of the hospital industry.
- A state or local health authority is created to issue the bond. This authority must be the result of legislative action.
- Unlike other forms of government-backed financing, the authority does not acquire control of the assets once the debt has been paid. These lower equity restrictions make it feasible for hospitals to obtain funding, yet retain ownership.

- Repayment of the debt and interest is derived through the operations of the hospital, as opposed to relying on philanthropy and restricted funds.
- Interest rates on bonds are lower than other marketable securities because the lender does not have to pay federal income tax on the earnings. As an investment, the risk is low.
- The terms of the bonds are generally more favorable to hospitals than conventional financing. The term (i.e., number of years over which the bond must be paid off) can be extended, and there generally are provisions that allow assurance of further funding.

Although these trends and advantages have been helpful in facilitating hospital construction, renovation, and expansion, they have also made hospitals dependent on one major funding vehicle. This is a problem of vision. Hospital managers must be cognizant of the threats to tax-exempt bonds and should accordingly modify their long-run capital acquisition plans.

For the short run, assuming that tax-exempt revenue bonds will continue to be important as a funding mechanism for hospital construction, it is appropriate to understand how hospitals can make their bond offerings as marketable as possible. Laffey and Lappen examined this issue for all tax-exempt hospital bonds issued in 1974.[13] According to the results of their analysis, the most important factors that lower the net interest cost in a bond issue include debt service coverage and service area coverage. These findings are not surprising.

To the extent that a hospital is better positioned to cover debt through efficient operations leading to higher net income, it is able to lower the investment risk and possibly attain a higher bond rating. It is logical that the capability of a given service area or catchment area to provide sufficient numbers of admissions to maintain occupancy is a prerequisite to the marketability of a bond. When investors know that a hospital will be able to keep its beds filled with paying customers, they are less worried that hospital construction will result in unfilled, idle beds that raise costs and threaten the ability to service the debt.

Bond Ratings

Familiarity with the terminology surrounding bonds is essential in view of the prevalence of this financing mechanism among health care organizations. Not all bonds are rated equally, but according to their yield and risk. A health care organization wants to offer bonds with the highest rating because there are significant implications for the interest rate that will be paid for the borrowed capital. Nurse administrators may not be directly involved in establishing a bond rating or deriving funding through bonds for hospital construction. Nonetheless, they should understand why their organization has a lower rating than another organization and what that lower bond rating implies operationally.

The financial market comprises millions of investors who somehow must be able to communicate effectively about a bond (whether tax-exempt or not) and its ability to provide a return on investment. Investors recognize that generally the higher the risk of a bond, the higher will be the yield (i.e., the interest rate) until the bond attains its full maturity (i.e., is fully paid for). To facilitate the sale of bonds a convention must be developed that conveys the financial parameters surrounding a bond issue. Such a convention has been created by reputable investment services in the form of bond ratings. These firms assess the attractiveness of the bond and its inherent risk. As a result a bond is graded, and investors can use the information to compare one bond with another. This comparative rating is the standard for understanding whether a hospital's bond is a risky investment or whether there is low risk.

Two rating services have gained distinction for their assessment of bonds. Standard & Poor's Corporation and Moody's Investor Services are recognized as reliable authorities in the area of bond ratings. Some of their gradings are illustrated as follows:

Degree of Risk	Yield	Standard & Poor's Corporation Rating	Interpretation	Moody's Investor Services Rating	Interpretation
Low	Low	AAA	Highest rating	Aaa	Best quality
•	•	AA	High grade	Aa	High quality
•	•	•		•	
•		BBB	Medium grade	Baa	Lower medium
Medium	Medium	•		•	grade
•		•		•	
•	•	•		•	
•	•	B	Speculative	B	Generally lacks
•	•	•		•	characteristics
•	•	•		•	of a desirable
•	•	•		•	investment
•	•	CC	Outright	Ca	Speculative to
•	•	•	Speculation	•	a high degree
•	•	•		•	
High	High	D	In default	C	Lowest grade

The rating is just a starting point from which an investment should be analyzed. Within a given rating category there may be substantial variance in how much risk or yield a given bond has been assessed. Remember that the risk and yield relationship is only a generalization. Over the entire course of the financial market we have seen that bonds with a higher risk provide a higher yield, but there are exceptions that invalidate this conclusion.

Investment agencies often use the following criteria when assessing the bond rating for a particular issue:[14]

- Peak debt historical coverage
- Peak debt first-year coverage
- Cash flow change
- Net working capital to sales
- Debt per bed
- Beginning beds
- Relative occupancy
- Percentage of Medicaid revenue
- Market share
- Expense per patient day

According to Cleverley and Nutt these criteria act to benefit larger health care organizations.[15] A large organization is needed to attain the economies of scale to produce favorable ratings on the specified criteria. They also observe that third party payment often works against the attainment of these criteria.

The hospital field has historically not offered bonds that could be classified as the highest rating or the best quality. Most bond offerings fall in the A+ (21 percent), A (upper medium grade) (41 percent), A− (15 percent) or BBB (18 percent) range on the Standard & Poor's index.[16] The reasons for this are primarily related to risks. Earlier, we stated that hospitals were relatively low risk investments. Yet, because hospitals are dependent on third party payers for their revenue, the amount of revenue can be controlled by only a handful of payers. This presents risk to the hospital, particularly in view of prospective payment. Hospitals are also limited in their production capacity because they cannot extend inpatient services beyond 100 percent occupancy (although greater productivity can be achieved through outpatient services). They are constrained in their ability to raise levels of production. Construction of new beds is usually controlled by state and local health planning agencies through the certificate of need laws. Moreover the industry is already perceived to be overbedded. Add to these factors high medical malpractice risks associated with inpatient care and it becomes increasingly apparent that hospitals do present a significant degree of risk as far as an investment is concerned.

Another way for financial analysts in the health field to assess bond ratings is to associate the ratings with some of the common operating characteristics of hospitals. This is especially relevant because the factors are often tangible variables that their hospitals can control. Nurse administrators and their departments can influence the value of these variables. For example, they can diligently achieve cost control in nursing programs or departments and thereby increase the operating margin of a hospital. A higher operating margin in turn can be translated into a higher bond rating.

This association between bond rating and generic hospital characteristics has been studied by Hee and Henkel.[17] Their conclusions regarding the association can be summarized in this manner:

Hospital Characteristic	Association between Characteristic and Bond Rating
Number of Beds	Positive
Gross Revenues	Positive
Operating Margin	Positive
Ability To Service Debt	Positive
Percent of Long-Term Debt of Capital	Negative
Debt Service to Patient Day	Negative

According to these results, as a hospital has a higher number of beds and higher gross revenues, its bond rating is apt to be higher. Clearly the larger institution gives the appearance of being less threatened by the environment it inhabits.

The empirical association between the hospital characteristics and bond ratings generally could be predicted as a result of sound management practices. When a hospital has a solid operating margin (i.e., profitability), it has a high bond rating. A solid operating margin implies a better capacity to service debt (i.e., make principal and interest payments), which in turn contributes to a higher bond rating. In contrast, when a hospital has a high percentage of long-term debt to total capital, or when the average debt that must be serviced per patient day is high, the hospital is in a more precarious financial position. The result is a lower bond rating (indicated by a negative association). From these empirical results, nurse administrators should understand that there is no mystical way to derive a high bond rating.[18] Attention to conservative financial management of a hospital is more likely to lead to a high bond rating than any other factor.

PROGNOSIS FOR FUTURE FINANCING

What is the prognosis for future financing given the fact that the major source of funds for hospital construction—tax-exempt revenue bonds—are under attack? This is an important question because the capacity of the hospital field to maintain productive assets is affected by its sources of capital. Surprisingly, what had once been a very optimistic picture for the health field as far as the capital base has progressively become more dismal over the last two decades. This is a result of at least two major forces—regulation and reimbursement. Not only has it become more difficult to acquire the right to build or renovate facilities, it has also been more difficult to be properly reimbursed for invested capital.[19] Will these trends continue in the future?

In order for nurse administrators to appreciate the trends in hospital financing and the implication for the future, it is necessary to review the various philosophies about capital issues in the hospital field. A rich history of predictions about a hospital capital crisis has often been overlooked by hospital executives. Why this has occurred is uncertain. It may be that hospitals have been so involved with operational issues that these broader issues have been left unattended. Consequently their alternatives are increasingly constrained.

Early Warnings

In the 1960s there was growing interest in how hospitals would meet their capital needs in the future. At that time there were decreases in government grants and appropriations as well as philanthropy. The impact of these trends was the reduction of the basis for capitalization. Faced with 20- to 30-year investments for new plant and equipment, many hospitals began to see that their ability to obtain financing was growing more limited. Few contemplated how difficult capitalization would be in the future.

At this time there were essentially three methods of financing future hospital capital needs:[20]

1. Obtain contributions from philanthropy on either a specific donor or mass fund-raising basis.
2. Borrow capital from the financial markets and use revenue to service debt and interest payments.
3. Plan for the future by accumulating earnings in a pool of retained earnings or by using depreciation to create a reserve for capital.

The first two options are not novel as far as recommendations for funding future capital needs. It is the last suggestion of using depreciation that was a departure from traditional hospital management practices.

Depreciation refers to the deterioration or "wearing out" of plant and equipment through use. Depreciation is a normal cost of doing business and is treated as an expense. Yet depreciation does not result in any out-of-pocket expenditures in a given accounting period. It can create a valuable hidden surplus if an organization undertakes a conservative management of the expense. Revenues must be sufficient to balance the expense of depreciation. There is, however, no direct expenditure of those funds. For most organizations it is a temptation to translate this as a surplus for operating expenditures. By setting aside a reserve fund for depreciation expense, they would gradually build up a retained surplus available to replace obsolescent assets.

The main flaw in this strategy is the fact that assets are usually kept on the books at historical cost. This historical cost does not represent the current cost of replacing those assets at existing market rates. A hospital that was built five years ago may have a historical cost of $13.4 million. Its replacement could easily exceed $19 million today due to inflation in costs of materials and construction. The best way to compensate for this depletion is to use accelerated depreciation. However, a controversy ensued between hospitals and third party payers as to which methods of accounting for depreciation were legitimate.

The question of which depreciation method to employ is an important one, but perhaps it is not as important as retaining earnings. Health facilities need to create a reserve to fund new construction, replacement, renovation, or expansion. Very few hospitals heeded these warnings. The reimbursement climate may have been an important factor affecting the financial management posture in the health care field at this time. Consequently, hospitals overlooked their plans for investment and derived serious shortfalls in replacement funds.

Growing Evidence of Funding Problems

It became increasingly apparent in the 1970s that hospital reimbursement from third party payers was not keeping pace with inflation in construction costs. At least two major factors were contributing to this growing dilemma.[21] On one hand third party reimbursers such as Medicare were supportive of covering operating expenses related to patient care, depreciation, and interest costs from debt. They did not, however, cover the costs of bad debts or free care. These costs were often subsidized by other third party payers or by private paying patients. Hospitals covered the current operations expenses by using funds that normally would be retained for replacement of capital assets.

The predominantly nonprofit nature of the hospital industry also contributed to the capital replacement dilemma.[22] Nonprofit hospitals could not legally make a profit, and they could not be reimbursed for bad debts and charity care. As a result they could not generate internal funds to cover the cost of new capital. A growing tension developed between third party payers and hospitals. The outcome was also a growing deterioration of hospital plant and equipment because necessary funding was not available.

Proof of the funding problems was empirically substantiated by Cleverley, who foresaw a continuing erosion of the capital base of hospitals if the cost-based reimbursement formula were continued.[23] According to Cleverley's analysis, it would take more than total cost-based reimbursement to resolve the dilemma because of the inflation costs confronting new capital investment. A workable solution would require that depreciation costs (funded under most third party payers such as Medicare) be adjusted to reflect current inflationary costs. This price adjustment would then help hospitals accumulate capital at a rate greater than the adjusted historical cost-based depreciation.

The Capital Crisis

By the 1980s the problem confronting hospitals in funding capital investment had increased substantially. Some simple factors convey the growing crisis in the capital position of hospitals:[24]

	Capital Asset (Billions)	Depreciation Necessary To Fund Replacement (Billions)	Inflation Deficit (Billions)
1980 Hospital Asset Historical Base	$68.2	$20.4	
Adjustment for: Consumer Price Level Inflation	$123.3	$46.4	$26.0
Construction Cost Inflation	$125.7	$49.5	$29.5
Technology Inflation	$150.4	$68.2	$48.2

According to these estimates, the 1980 hospital asset base of $68.2 billion on historical basis would require $20.4 billion of funded depreciation to prudently cover replacement costs of new hospital assets. This does not accurately portray the actual funds needed to replace assets. To the historical base must be added $55.1 billion for consumer price level inflation, $2.4 billion for construction cost inflation, and $24.7 billion for the technological costs of hospital assets. Thus, the estimated hospital base is $150.4 billion; a figure that requires $68.2 billion to fund depreciation. This is $48.2 billion more than that provided through Medicare's reimbursement provisions.

In other words, hospitals need an additional $48.2 billion to cover the replacement of existing hospital assets. Where these funds can be obtained is the primary question confronting hospitals. Realistically it is unreasonable to expect that hospitals will fund this deficit out of retained earnings, given the history of limited planning for future asset replacement. Third party reimbursement is also a dubious choice, since third party revenues are projected to decrease rather than increase. Prospective payment may only exacerbate the situation rather than resolve it. Philanthropy and government appropriations are also unlikely sources since they are gradually shrinking.

One viable method for hospitals to obtain capital appears to be diversification into new lines of service.[25,26] Diversification should be lucrative enough that surplus income would pay for new principal and interest payments from long-term debt or bond premiums. In many cases this would necessitate restructuring hospitals into complex organizations where the acute care component was only one portion. This would allow retention of tax-exempt status and maintenance of requirements for third party reimbursement. Subsidiary divisions could use hospital assets to make a profit, which in turn is given back to the hospital in the form of a rent payment (in the broad economic sense).

Diversification services are as broad as the imagination, resources, and population served allow. Hospitals are diversifying into home health care, surgicenters, mental health clinics, wellness programs, long-term care, primary care, alcohol and substance abuse treatment, diagnostic centers, and other clever noninpatient endeavors. Hospitals need to be innovative in how they define their services and in how they use this redefinition to resolve the capital crisis.

Another vehicle for resolving the capital crisis is to seek corporate status. Many nonprofit hospitals have been reshaping their set of organizational goals by selling their assets to for-profit corporations. These corporations have been able to fund capital investments through equity markets. The concept is the same as that for any other form of business. Incorporation and stock offering allows a hospital (chain) to acquire capital. There are serious and substantial tax implications from investor ownership. But, when confronted by the capital acquisition problem, it is apparent that many hospitals will be forced to pursue rather drastic measures.

In sum, the prognosis for future capitalization in the health care field appears to be rather dismal. Hospitals have a history of neglecting the financial planning function. They are now confronted by a problem of serious proportions, yet they have few reserves available to fund the replacement of existing plant and equipment. This occurs in an environment where third party payments are increasingly restricted and where costs are rising. On the surface there may appear to be few alternatives available. However, it is precisely this sort of challenge that has traditionally brought out the best in health care and business managers. More likely than not it is this ingenuity that will be exercised in order for hospitals to survive.

Unless some drastic changes are made in the very near future in third party payments, the hospital field will continue to gravitate toward a more businesslike orientation. For those people who philosophically believe in the nonprofit nature of health care, such transition may be intolerable. However, this question must also be balanced by the capital needs of the industry. In the long run, economic realities will undoubtedly determine the precise nature of capital issues of hospitals and other health care organizations.

FEASIBILITY STUDIES

The prognosis for future financing of capital assets in the health field suggests that health care managers will become more analytical in their capital investments. The immediate by-product of this analysis is the financial feasibility study. Although most feasibility studies are designed to qualify a hospital for bond funding, feasibility studies are also useful in assessing many other capital expenditures.[27,28] The results can be used both internally and externally. Internal users such as top management and the board of directors can ascertain whether demand is sufficient for a project and what revenue projections will likely accompany varying demand levels. External users such as bond rating agencies, investors, underwriters, and government agencies will analyze the reports to determine the desirability of funding projects according to their own purposes and goals.[29]

Forecasting accuracy is the key to a successful feasibility study.[30] Without accurate estimates of demand and the impact of revenues and expenses, the feasibility study will not make a meaningful contribution. Therefore, the forecasts serve as the foundation for the remaining components of the feasibility study. A financial feasibility study should consist of the following stages:[31]

- Demand Phase
  —Internal Analysis
  —External Analysis
  —Facility Forecasts
  —Ancillary Service Forecasts
- Revenue and Expense Impact
  —Staffing Levels
  —Staffing Expenses
  —Nonsalary Expenses
  —Gross Revenues
- Capital Transactions
  —Existing Assets
    Replacement Assets
  —Proposed Project

The preceding stages represent a general model only. Each funding project has unique characteristics that justify altering this model to meet specific assessment needs.

Financial feasibility studies are usually prepared with the help of consultants for major investments. There is a perception that an external consultant will add objectivity to the analysis. This may be appropriate for some, but certainly not all, projects. Often existing managerial staff can prepare the feasibility study—nurse administrators are ideal candidates for inclusion in this process. The goal is to provide as accurate an estimate as possible of the outcomes from investing capital.

COST OF CAPITAL

An organization's cost of capital is the rate of return that must be earned on a capital investment to maintain the economic value of the health care institution. In investor-owned organizations, the cost of capital is the return demanded by investors in the securities (e.g., stock) offered by the corporation. Economic value or rate of return is essential to market services. Ability to survive financially over the long run is associated with the capacity to pay the desired (i.e., market) rate of return. If a health care organization continually makes investments (i.e., in programs, services, equipment, or facilities) that do not earn a rate of return at least equal to its cost of capital, it cannot survive unless subsidized by an external funding source or interest group.

Assume that an investor-owned hospital presents the following profile for its sources of capital:[32]

Source of Capital	% Contribution		Estimated Cost Source		Average Cost
Stock	.60	×	.16	−	.096
Debt	.24	×	.125	=	.030
Retained Earnings	.16	×	.10	=	.016
			Average Cost =		.142

Note that the average cost of capital—of obtaining funds to invest in capital assets—for the investor-owned hospital is 14.2 percent. The precise cost of each source depends on several factors. In the case of stock, the cost of this capital is related to the market-determined risk. The cost of debt is ascertained from the interest payments for long-term obligations. Meanwhile, the cost of retained earnings is calculated from the interest payments that are received from investment of the funds in the marketable securities or demand deposits (shown above as 10 percent—a feasible rate for a certificate of deposit).

Determining the cost of capital for a health care organization is a complex task. Many approaches can be used, but they all require a fairly advanced knowledge of financial methods. For nurse administrators, it is sufficient to recognize that calculations of the cost of capital are usually undertaken to define the minimum threshold for acceptable return on new investments. Therefore, if nurse administrators are participating in a program feasibility study, they may wish to compute the cost of capital to determine whether the proposed project produces a return above the organization's cost of capital. Assistance from the chief financial officer or financial staff is likely to be needed in the actual calculations. By undertaking this analysis, one more valuable piece of information is acquired with which to evaluate capital investments.

NOTES

1. Ross Mullner et al., "Debt Financing: An Alternative for Hospital Construction Funding," *Healthcare Financial Review* 13 (April 1983): 18–24.

2. M. Lightle, "Changes in the Sources of Capital," *Hospital Financial Management* 11 (February 1981): 42–47.

3. Mullner et al., "Debt Financing."

4. W. Thomas Berriman, William G. Essick, and Peter I. Bertivanga, "Public Sources of Long Term Financing," *Topics in Health Care Financing* 2 (Winter 1975): 7.

5. Walter K. Palmer, "Financing Capital in a Hospital-based Prepayment Plan," *Hospital Financial Management* 11 (December 1981): 62–66.

6. Hugh W. Long, "Investment Decision Making in the Health Care Industry: The Future," *Health Services Research* 14 (Fall 1979): 183–206.

7. Mullner et al., "Debt Financing."

8. Jack R. Schlosser, "Venture Capital: Past, Present, and Future Applications," *Topics in Health Care Financing* 11 (Winter 1984): 63–71.

9. Robert H. Rosenfield, "Tax-exempt Hospitals Explore New Ways to Attract Equity," *Hospital Financial Management* 35 (October 1981): 59–61.

10. Victor E. Schimmel and Joan M. Annett, "Capital Financing for Ambulatory Care Facilities," *Journal of Ambulatory Care Management* 7 (November 1984): 4–17.

11. Mullner et al., "Debt Financing."

12. "Refinancing and Refunding Options," *Topics in Health Care Financing* 5 (Fall 1978): 43–53.

13. William J. Laffey and Stan Lappen, "Tax-exempt Hospital Financing: Revenue Bonds," *Health Care Management Review* (Fall 1976): 19–30.

14. D. Cain and R. Gilbert, "Credit Rating Agencies and Hospital Lenders," *Topics in Health Care Financing* 5 (Fall 1978): 55–64.

15. William O. Cleverley and Paul C. Nutt, "Credit Evaluation of Hospitals," *Topics in Health Care Financing* (Summer 1981): 81–86.

16. William P. Condon, "Hospital Revenue Bonds—How They're Rated," *Hospital Financial Management* 35 (September 1981): 60, 62, 64.

17. Dickson L. Hee and Author J. Henkel, "Operational Statistics and Bond Ratings," *Healthcare Financial Management* 13 (October 1983): 52–56.

18. John E. Gilchrist and Eileen S. Winterble, "Getting Through a Debt Rating," *Hospital Financial Management* 12 (April 1982): 58–61.

19. William O. Cleverley, "Reimbursement for Capital Costs," *Topics in Health Care Financing* 6 (Fall 1979): 127–139.

20. Ettore Barbatelli, "Using Depreciation to Provide for Future Hospital Financial Needs," *Hospitals,* July 16, 1976, pp. 46–49.

21. Edward L. Walls, "Hospital Dependency on Long-term Debt," *Financial Management* 1 (Spring 1972): 42–47.

22. Ronald Copeland and Philip Jacobs, "Cost of Capital, Target Rate of Return, and Investment Decision Making," *Health Services Research* 16 (Fall 1981): 335–341.

23. William O. Cleverley, "Is Hospital Capital Being Eroded under Cost Reimbursement?" *Hospital Administration* 19 (Summer 1974): 58–73.

24. Charles Bradford, George Caldwell, and Jeff C. Goldsmith, "The Hospital Capital Crisis," *Harvard Business Review* 60 (September-October 1982): 56–68.

25. Howard L. Smith and Richard A. Reid, *Competitive Hospitals* (Rockville, Md.: Aspen Publishers, 1986).

26. Jeff C. Goldsmith, "The Health Care Market: Can Hospitals Survive?" *Harvard Business Review* 58 (September-October 1980): 100.

27. "The Role of the Independent Financial Feasibility Study," *Topics in Health Care Financing* 5 (Fall 1978): 73–80.

28. Frances M. Hoffman, "Developing Capital Expenditure Proposals," *Journal of Nursing Administration* 15 (September 1985): 32–34.

29. Warren Quinley, "Hospital Feasibility Studies: Are They Management Tools or Required Nuisances?" *Hospital Financial Management* 36 (October 1982): 50, 52, 54.

30. John M. Aderholdt, "Forecasting Accuracy: A Valuable Key to Financial Feasibility Studies for Hospitals," *Hospital Financial Management* 35 (September 1981): 52–54, 57–58, 60.

31. Peter W. Bruton, "Preparing for Financial Feasibility Study," *Healthcare Financial Management* 37 (May 1983): 87–88.

32. Bruce R. Newmann, James D. Suver, and William N. Zelman, *Financial management: Concepts and applications for health care providers* (United States: Rynd Communications, 1984).

Chapter 10

A Nursing Perspective on Financial Management

What is the outlook for financial management practices in nursing? This question may have stimulated little interest before the 1980s, but the health care environment has changed so radically that the question deserves serious consideration. Many alterations in third party reimbursement and in the health care marketplace have had a profound impact on the roles of health care professionals. Nursing is one of the areas in which this impact has opened significant opportunities and responsibilities. The issue is whether nurses will recognize these opportunities and take advantage of them.

PRESSURES FROM THE HEALTH CARE ENVIRONMENT

A primary problem with prospective payment and competition is that their effects do not remain at an organizational level. They eventually filter down throughout all managerial, supervisory, and clinical levels. In the ensuing confusion, what appears to be a programmatic or departmental problem (e.g., nursing staff turnover) may actually be the impact of prospective payment, or the influence of competition. Once cause and effect become confused, it is increasingly difficult to design and implement the sort of management interventions that address prospective payment constraints or competitive demands. Nursing administrators need to analyze exactly how these pressures filter down throughout a health care organization. By understanding this effect, they will be better prepared to construct lasting solutions to these problems. The result should be an important contribution to the bottom line as well as the attainment of primary nursing goals.

Nursing administrators are responsible for forging organizational responses to pressures generated by the health care environment. This is not an easy assignment, but as Aaron Levenstein has noted, "To the timid, the need for making new adjustments is always alarming. The true professional will not shrink from challenge; on the contrary he craves it. Crisis presents an opportunity for change, and change holds out the possibility of progress."[1] Nursing administrators are not alone in responding to environmental pressures such as prospective payment and competition; *all* nursing staff are responsible albeit in varying degrees.[2,3] Table 10–1 summarizes this variability in response.

Competition

A primary result of prospective payment and competition is a series of constraints on the ability of nursing units, programs, and departments to perform at their highest level. Not only are health care organizations concerned with controlling costs, they also must pay attention to the marketability of their services. In many cases this implies that a greater investment will have to be made in promotional programs that raise costs. In other instances an entirely new strategy may have to be adopted to provide high quality and low cost care.

For example, hospitals have begun to diversify into many related health services. The freestanding community hospital today is much more consumer oriented and has developed an extensive component of new programs. Urgent care, home care, wellness programs, hospice care, and other alternatives are being considered

Table 10–1 A Continuum of Nursing Responses to the Health Care Environment

Organizational Level	Responsibilities for Managing Environmental Pressures
Clinical Staff Nurse	1. Develop and maintain a general awareness of the economic and fiscal environments
	2. Develop and maintain a general awareness of changes in national health policy and implications for *direct* patient care
Head Nurse/Supervisor	1. Promote, educate, and interpret environmental issues
	2. Translate stresses of fiscal constraints on clinical staff to upper management
	3. Translate necessity of required changes from upper management to clinicians
Nursing Administrator	1. Design programs for nursing care based on economic and social efficiency as well as clinical effectiveness
	2. Provide expertise in enacting organizational structure and design
	3. Balance the intensifying conflict between cost containment and clinical capabilities

and applied by hospitals that are interested in circumventing the negative impact of competition.

The growth of new programs has significant meaning for nurses. Every new program must be justified before investments are made. Health care organizations are interested in new programs because of their ability to provide a higher return on investment than existing programs and services.[4,5] This is a bottom-line orientation that is receiving extensive support in the health care field. The issue before nurses and nurse administrators is the extent to which they will become proficient in developing or running programs that offer a good return on investment.

Nursing program proposals must demonstrate long-run profitability *in addition to* contributing to marketability, quality of care, and the support of existing services. Financial feasibility is a critical criterion in these new program alternatives. Furthermore, existing programs will be scrutinized to determine whether they offer services efficiently and effectively. Health care organizations must control or drive down their costs if revenues do not increase. Nursing programs will be asked to do more than their share because the costs of nursing care represent a substantial percentage of the budget.

Prospective Payment

Budgetary restrictions arising from prospective payment result in general belt-tightening. Consequently, nurse administrators cannot simply introduce innovative programs and services that help their organizations respond to competition or that effectively institute a program of cost control. Budgetary restrictions force nursing programs and departments to produce more services with less resources. Nurse administrators must somehow encourage their staff members to be more productive despite decreases in benefits, compensation, rewards, and staffing levels. This management plan may be very difficult to implement.

More incremental planning is generally undertaken by top management as it seeks to articulate a competitive strategy or to devise a working program of cost control. There are more false starts on new programs because the precise impact of either competition or prospective payment has not been ascertained. Hence there is uncertainty about which directions to pursue. Structurally the organization changes as efforts are made to provide the highest level of support to programs constituting the competitive edge. Nursing programs are often requested to provide services that support this competitive advantage. This in turn alters reporting relationships and necessitates consolidation of work units, programs, and departments.

Programs and services that do not directly contribute to the strategic plan or are not cost-effective are often terminated. Nursing programs that support health care and are nonrevenue generating (e.g., health education, wellness clinics, and so forth) are frequently terminated in order to control costs. This tendency to cut financially weak programs is consistent with prevalent responses to prospective payment and competition. Nurse administrators ultimately must achieve these performance targets with the same or often with fewer resources. However, there are limitations to the creativity that can be invoked to resolve these pressures.

ORGANIZATIONAL RESPONSES TO THE PRESSURES

These and other side effects represent the consequences from higher competition and shifts toward prospective pricing. The health care organization must respond. It has two basic choices. One is to fine-tune internal operations, which results in the filtering phenomenon noted above. The second alternative involves strategic management changes that influence the mission, goals, and resources of an organization. Depending on their level in the hierarchy, nurse administrators will probably be involved in the efforts to optimize service delivery. They must not lose the perspective that this contribution has significant financial ramifications. It is the successive aggregation of cost containment across all services that ultimately provides financially respectable operations.

Filtering Problems

Nurse administrators may question why competition and prospective payment should have such an in-depth effect that they ultimately threaten the performance of a health care organization. A primary factor that causes the filtering phenomenon is inexperience of health care organizations in managing competition. Very little is really known about what strategies to pursue because most health facilities and providers have never faced overt competition. Consequently, top management thrashes about a great deal in trying out one strategy and then revising it or substituting another. This is quite apparent in the area of hospital diversification. There is a high degree of uncertainty associated with making a commitment to a specific plan of action. However in the final analysis, virtually any diversification alternative appears acceptable.

In addition to inexperience in managing competition, health care organizations have been unable to create necessary internal buffers rapidly. These buffers could protect the operating level from the adverse side effects of prospective pricing and competition. For example, nursing homes that are competing for private pay patients are usually so heavily invested in upgrading the appearance of their facilities and adding fine touches to their services that they are understaffed. Increasingly these organizations are managed on a shoestring with department heads such as nursing directors experiencing the direct impact of the resource constraints. Stretched to the limit, the director of nursing has less time to protect staff nurses who are asked to produce beyond the level appropriate for the compensation they receive or the conditions under which they work. In sum, a vicious cycle ensues in the resource–constrained situation. Nurse administrators are unable to resolve problems because resources are not available (e.g., nursing staff) to maintain service delivery.

Both prospective payment and competition filter down throughout health care organizations to the essence of service delivery. The nurse manager is the person responsible for protecting staff members from the adverse effects of these pressures. Yet their ability is constrained because resources (e.g., allocations to marketing, upgrading the physical plant, or start-up of new services) are being used to support hospital-wide marketing programs. Ingenuity can supplement the lack of resources, but eventually even creativity cannot substitute for needed resources such as more staff or supplies.

The nurse administrator may receive little help from top management because of the inexperience of the upper echelons in managing competition and prospective payment. There may be very little assistance or guidance available from top management. The impression is that the fight against competition and prospective payment is being subsidized by the operating levels, particularly nursing services.

Protecting Key Services

Although top management may not be totally adept at preventing the negative effects of competition from reaching the nursing level, this is not an excuse for nurse administrators to let these factors adversely influence their staff members.[6] The first step is to understand what protection is needed and how it can be implemented. This is the essence of leadership—to prevent distracting factors from filtering down from other organizational levels or from outside the organization.

When external pressures affect staff members by distracting them from their immediate responsibilities, the efficiency and effectiveness of a nursing unit, program, or department may suffer. For example, protection is needed for the critical care nurse who is responsible for too many patients when staffing levels have been reduced as a result of decreased occupancy and a competitor's successful marketing campaign.

Innovative techniques might incorporate any number of useful management tactics. Nursing administrators can set financially oriented goals and objectives for staff that relate to specific tasks associated with the nursing unit, program, or department. At the same time they should avoid allocating staff time to tasks associated with nonprogram agendas. In line with the objective-setting process, nurse administrators should reward performance that achieves prespecified goals and objectives rather than performance that achieves crisis-generated goals and objectives.

Nurse administrators should contemplate working with other managers to articulate plans and define budget targets for their programs. They should avoid letting others define goals and objectives for their program without direct input. The nurse administrator must maintain control and function as the authority responsible for assigning tasks rather than let others make such assignments. Alternatively, it may be appropriate to document the need for additional resources (e.g., more staff, new equipment, or added supplies) that are necessary in order to meet new expectations.

Nurse administrators can also analytically determine the impact of prospective payment and competition, which influences the ability of their programs to attain prespecified levels of performance. For example, the level of resources required to complete a given goal may be more than the resources allocated. This difference between resources allocated and service expectations must be communicated clearly yet forcefully to upper management. In other situations it may be necessary to alert other managers when they disrupt the performance of the nursing unit, program, or department by intervening in the structure and process of those services. Nurse administrators need to underscore the integrity of their authority.

Setting Financial Standards

It should be apparent to nursing administrators that staff members define their work goals in concert with the goals and attitudes created by their supervisor. Even for the most ambitious or intrinsically motivated nurse, the prevailing climate of the program or department can alter commitment to goal accomplishment. The nurse administrator's role, therefore, is to help guide a group of nurses toward high productivity, lower costs, quality care, and overall financial respectability. Above all, the nurse administrator must ensure that it is not staff nurses who are setting productivity, cost control, or quality goals. The managerial challenge is to motivate and direct nurses toward higher levels of performance.[7] If this approach is not undertaken, targeted objectives that were established in the budgeting process may go unmet.

With higher levels of competition and the growth of prospective payment, it is inevitable that nurse administrators will ask their staff members to perform at higher levels to improve financial performance. In order to be competitive and hence financially successful, a health care organization must produce a higher quality and lower cost service. Every organizational level is concerned with this response because aggregate performance eventually determines whether an organization has the financial resources to survive. While there are staff members (e.g., physicians and nurses) who can influence the aggregate service at a proportionally higher rate than other staff members (e.g., housekeeping staff, laboratory technicians, food service aides, and so forth), it is nonetheless true that *every* person can influence the overall product or service.

Health care managers are responsible for directing employees toward higher levels of financial performance despite less than favorable conditions. Although a health care organization may require higher quality and lower cost services, this does not necessarily imply that it will have the resources to reward nurses who achieve exemplary performance. In fact, the reverse may actually be true. Competition places an added strain that may threaten the resource base. More dollars have to be allocated to promotional efforts such as advertising. The profile that emerges is one of ever-increasing austerity for the operating level. One managerial resolution to this problem is to set higher expectations. Although these expectations may not always be met, the process does point personnel in the right direction.

Coping with Change

The structure and authority relationships of health care organizations confronting prospective payment and competition will experience change. The key for nurse administrators is to help their staff members cope with this change while at the same time not jeopardizing financial goals of the nursing program or department. Nurse administrators can play an active role in helping subordinates cope with new policies, procedures, and reporting relationships that emanate from demands for improved financial performance.

Nurse administrators need to instill the idea that a specific nursing unit, program, or department is only a means for the organization to accomplish its specific ends. One of these is financial solvency. Although the nursing staff may be comfortable with its performance, the staff must proceed with the best interests of the organization in mind. This may mean suboptimizing inputs in the delivery of care in order to derive better overall performance by the health care organization. For example, a nurse practitioner may be asked to decrease the amount of time spent with patients in order to raise the number of patients seen per hour. This request attempts to maximize financial performance through higher productivity. From the nurse's perspective it severely threatens the nurse practitioner/patient relationship. But the change in operating procedure is necessary if the organization is to pursue ever-increasing efficiency and hence profitability.

Nurse administrators need to establish their programs as champions of cooperation. This means that the nursing department acquires an identity of willingness to cooperate. Given the turmoil surrounding prospective payment and competition, a positive outlook is vitally needed; this will make the organization's response to pressures that threaten financial viability much easier. For example, once it is apparent that a budget will have to be cut, nursing staff members lost, a new unit manager introduced, or other similar changes induced by prospective payment and competition, nurse administrators must help move staff beyond dysfunctional grief and regret toward productivity in a new context.

Advocates for Nurses

With the impact of competition and prospective payment nurse administrators will experience the uncomfortable fact that their budgets are shrinking or at least not growing as fast as they had in the past. This places a nursing unit, program, or department in direct conflict with the total health care organization. On one hand, it is essential that nursing programs share in the restraints imposed by reimbursement and competition. On the other hand, it is critical that nursing programs continue to pursue plans for development, growth, and excellence in performance. The contention that develops between nursing program and organizational goals is not easy to resolve because it may be necessary for programs to subordinate their interests (or achieve suboptimization) in order that the overall organization's effort is optimized.

The consequence of this conflict between program and organization is clearly seen at budget time. Whether it is during the budgeting process or at another point when nursing programs or departments are being asked to sacrifice, nurse administrators must act as advocates for their programs. It is essential that nurse administrators build a strong case and argue for the program in both informal and formal negotiations. If they do not accept this responsibility, who will? Nursing staff will recognize this failure. It will become exceptionally difficult to drive the department to excellent performance. The lesson for nurse administrators is easily understood: they must be the advocates for their program or department within the organizational infrastructure.

Activating Strategies for Managing External Pressures

Health care organizations are facing a new environment that requires an experienced and businesslike approach to operations. Unfortunately, most health care organizations and their nursing programs are not very well prepared to respond to this challenge because, despite their best intentions, they have never had to confront the constraints presented by many factors in this new environment. Although the top management staff is primarily responsible for developing new strategies and tactics to resolve the challenges of these constraints, it appears that the actual methods for altering daily operations will have to come from the operational level. Nurse administrators will ultimately be responsible for translating the constraints of prospective payment, competition, and similar external pressures into workable solutions.

External pressures such as these present an exciting opportunity for nursing administrators if they are willing and able to rise to the challenge. Whether it is through protecting the nursing program and its staff members, setting higher financially oriented performance standards, maintaining a propensity to cope with change, or acting as an advocate for a program, many management strategies may be invoked by nurse administrators to respond to external forces. Such strategies are predicated on nurse administrators creating new responses consistent with overall organizational strategies and also consistent with the improvement of nursing program performance. In the end it is the ability to help the organization achieve its goals that is critical for nursing units, programs, and departments.

STRATEGIES FOR FINANCIAL MANAGEMENT

The strategies defined above are most useful in adapting a health care organization and its respective nursing programs to general external pressures from factors such as prospective payment, competition, retrenchment, and changing public attitudes toward health care. The problem for nurse managers is to develop responses that prevent these pressures from adversely influencing the financial performance of nursing units, programs, or departments.

Nurse administrators will discover that an exceptional number of financial management strategies can be integrated within a general philosophy or perspective on controlling operations. Strategic thinking is precisely the orientation that should be nurtured.

The development of a financial management perspective depends on broadening the nurse administrator's perspective. In this respect they must do the following:

- Become familiar with the terminology, concepts, and applications surrounding finance, yet incorporate these specific techniques within a general management approach.

- Integrate financial goals within their own perception of the objectives, goals, purpose, and mission of the nursing program and that of the health care organization.

- Integrate financial concerns in daily decision making. It is not enough to profess that a nursing program is committed to financial performance; such a commitment must be demonstrated in actual practice.

- Continue to study financial management concepts to improve their knowledge and ability to apply their skills. Central to this thought is personal discipline in acquiring information through professional journals, continuing education, and management development programs.

- Communicate to the upper echelon their preparation and willingness to assume greater responsibilities in financial issues related to nursing programs.

These and other basic steps are essential to nurse administrators if they wish to manage the financial aspects of performance from nursing programs.

A nurse administrator should have an understanding of specific strategies that will be implemented to help a program, department, or organization achieve better financial performance. There are several key concepts that underly such strategies. Nurse administrators need to move toward a strategic management perspective in order for their financial preparation to have full impact.

Monitoring Reimbursement Trends

A financially sensitive nurse administrator should be cognizant of all reimbursement trends if she/he intends to make a positive contribution to a program's performance. This may be the leading responsibility of all health services managers in today's environment. They must know where reimbursement policies have been, what they currently are, and where they are headed in the future. Perhaps most critical is an awareness of future directions. It is easy to determine where health care reimbursement policy is at any given moment simply by reading and digesting the existing regulations and policies. However, this activity may overlook many fine points that are valuable in planning future policies.

Far more critical is the ability to predict what a current reimbursement policy implies as far as opportunities and constraints. Once it is possible to correctly interpret the *implications* of reimbursement policy, it is then possible to adjust strategic and tactical plans. Remember that the strategic planning horizon is subject to major redirections in policy. Consequently, if the incorrect strategy is selected now, the organization may be forced to live with the strategy for longer than it wishes. Time is wasted in recognizing that a faulty strategy has been selected. A new strategy must be formed and then implemented to resolve the earlier misdirection. This situation results in less impressive financial performance.

For example, assume that a nonprofit nursing home decides that the capital portion of the state's Medicaid reimbursement policy will remain on a cost basis while the remaining portion is changed to prospective payment. Because of this incorrect assessment, the nursing home decides to plan the construction of a new 60-bed wing for three years hence, rather than immediately. The additional three years will be used to start a community fund drive serving as the primary capital base for the addition rather than using long-term debt to fund the construction. Furthermore, assume that the cost of borrowing capital rises rapidly over the next three years. Add to this hypothetical situation the eventuality that the capital portion did not remain on a cost basis but was included in the prospective portion the following year. What is the ultimate result?

The nurse administrator or other health care manager may have seriously misread the financial implications of this situation, thereby causing severe problems for the future. These problems are of immediate consequence:

- The nursing home has missed the opportunity to have its prospective rate include the costs of new construction. Since the prospective rate applies to all capital assets in the second year, and construction is planned to begin in the third year, the facility may not be reimbursed (or only partially reimbursed) for the capital expense.
- Higher interest costs are incurred because the construction was not begun when interest rates for borrowed capital were low.
- The facility is forced to rely on philanthropic contributions because the cost of long-term debt will not be fully covered.
- Other capital investments (e.g., in major equipment or refurbishing of existing plant) will be delayed while the nursing home sorts out the problems experienced with the new construction.

These are only a few of the problems that result when the strategic implications of reimbursement policies are misinterpreted.

Not every manager can correctly forecast the future. They are often reduced to guessing what direction a given policy will take over time. This is to be expected, and nurse administrators should be prepared for their own errors in interpreting policy changes in the health system. However, this does not absolve managers or minimize the frequency and magnitude of negative effects from incorrect assessments:

- More time should be allocated to those policies that have significant financial ramifications. It would be inappropriate to allocate substantial time to a decision on capital investment in a new piece of equipment and minimal time to monitoring reimbursement trends. The equipment will depreciate over a few years, while reimbursement is the essence of the organization's revenue base.
- Input should be obtained from knowledgeable sources both inside and outside the organization. It is essential to be exposed to many perspectives, but it is equally important to avoid an information overload. With respect to the circumstances surrounding any given health care organization, the management team has a much greater understanding of the impact of the surrounding environment than other so-called authorities.
- Reliance on popular trends or fads is often a result of a serious defect in management strategy.
- Financial viability should be the critical concern when interpreting a new or proposed policy. The manager must ascertain what each policy may imply for the financial well-being of the organization.

These thoughts are only a few of the guidelines that nurse administrators and other managers need to incorporate when interpreting and forecasting health policies.

By constantly asking what the financial impact of a policy will be on an organization, it may be possible to avoid seriously misinterpreting policy and hence devising an incorrect or practically inappropriate strategy.

The importance of monitoring reimbursement trends is amply demonstrated by the events surrounding Medicare's prospective payment system. Hospitals committed many errors of interpretation that dramatically influenced their selection of strategy. In the short run these errors decreased the ability to formulate effective strategies that supported, rather than detracted from, overall financial performance. Among these errors were the following:

- Hospitals focused too extensively on specific rates in each diagnostic related group. This was valuable in ensuring that correct reimbursement was obtained in each category, but the hospitals displaced their attention on an operational issue (i.e., specific rate determination) rather than on the strategic policy issues (i.e., control). Hospitals failed to realize quickly that if Medicare could control a specific rate in a specific diagnostic category, then it could also control total Medicare revenues.

- By focusing on specific rates and the mechanism for rate increases in the future, hospitals overlooked the fact that Medicare had effectively instituted a flat rate system; that is, it could set a rate in any given category and not raise it. The implication is that instead of a system of variable rates, Medicare or other third parties could eventually enforce a system of flat rates where revenue increases were limited.

- Hospitals became obsessed with their patient/payer mix. In other words, they formulated strategy around those payers that offered the most lucrative reimbursement for services. They did not perceive that even though some third parties were not adopting a diagnosis oriented payment scheme, they might instead be gravitating toward a much more restricted payment scheme founded on capitation or prepayment.

These are just a few of the misinterpretations prevalent in the health care field which occurred when Medicare's prospective payment system was implemented.

Nurse administrators should learn from these and similar experiences. Had hospitals maintained a focus on long-run financial implications rather than on short-run revenues they would have realized that the primary issue was rate control. With proper interpretation it might have been possible to formulate strategies that prepared health care organizations for a system of prepayment. Obviously such a system proposes entirely new financial requirements for both current operations as well as capital investment. These changes will continue to evolve in the future. For the present, it is essential to prevent further misdirections that might otherwise limit the strategic capability of health care organizations. In essence, both nurse administrators and their health care organizations need to become more adroit at monitoring and interpreting reimbursement trends.

Advancing Financial Excellence

At the heart of the new health care environment is the imperative for a comprehensive approach to performance. Past efforts were oriented to just one aspect of performance—quality of care. Now a new imperative is joined with the traditional performance goal. There is no question that health care organizations must achieve higher profitability. This applies to both for-profit and nonprofit institutions alike in the sense that a more efficiently run operation is needed, where costs do not grossly exceed revenues. The nurse administrator can play an important role in achieving these goals.

Foremost is the importance of advocating financial excellence through a performance orientation. Unless nurse administrators lead their staff toward better performance, who will? Support for excellence may not be the type normally envisioned by chief financial officers or financial managers in the sense that a direct, observable contribution is made to specific reductions of debt, expenses below budgeted limits, or cost savings. The incremental contribution made by nurse administrators in motivating personnel to produce more, to use fewer costly items in delivering services, or to help other programs and departments in their efforts to control costs or raise revenues illustrate commitment to financial excellence.

The nurse administrator's effort in advocating financial excellence will not be readily noted in prevailing financial statements or reports. The successes and victories of managing for financial excellence may be only partially reflected in: (1) a budget that is lower than the previous year, (2) fewer supply items consumed, (3) less use of a nursing registry or pool, or (4) personnel who consistently served patients without the extra full time staff equivalent that was vitally needed to prevent exhaustion among staff members. All of these victories seem insignificant and relatively inconsequential to the overall performance of the organization, yet this is where the foundation for good financial performance is constructed.

The nurse administrator's role in advocating financial excellence is not glamorous or highly visible. There is seldom a large-scale effort that the nurse administrator implements that results in the contribution to better performance. It is the successive accumulation of small victories that eventually culminates in better performance for the entire organization. This attitude and practice may be very difficult to create among nurse administrators because the reward systems of most organizations seldom compensate for such heroism or sacrifice. Nonetheless these end results are still vitally needed.

Negotiating with Top Management

A productive management strategy for nurse administrators who wish to promote the financial capability of their programs and departments is to work with top management rather than against it. Above all, nurse administrators want these negotiations to be two-way relationships. Without successful communication to the chief executive officer or the chief financial officer about the specific needs and end results of a viable nursing program, there is room for two significant errors. First, it is possible that top management will underestimate the needs of the nursing program. For example, the chief financial officer may decide when reviewing the master budget that the three requested full-time nursing staff members are not really essential for the next fiscal period. The nursing program loses the requested positions that may have been vital to the entire program.

Second, it is possible that top management will fail to communicate its precise interests to the nursing program. It is not unusual to discover significant misinterpretations in performance targets between management levels. It is unusual when a purposeful resolution is introduced to resolve these problems. Nurse administrators should be sensitive to these problems in view of the potential for more sophisticated reward and compensation systems in the future. Traditional reward systems have not been tied to performance. The result is that sometimes a program performs well and other times it does not.

Nurse administrators should work directly with top management (such as the chief financial officer and staff) in communicating plans and obtaining commitment to investments in nursing services. It is vital that the nurse administrator function as an advocate who is able to arrange proper support and who can validate a claim for further investment because it will ultimately pay off in terms of higher financial performance for the organization.

Becoming Financially Analytical

Although they are not directly responsible for providing documentation on proposed program changes, nurse administrators should be able to analyze financial implications from resource investments or from changes in service components. Too often nursing programs are asked to institute a change without examining the full consequences. In other situations there may be a deletion, substitution, or addition in staffing levels without thorough analysis.

These changes are made without in-depth analysis of financial consequences because nurse administrators are often ill-prepared either technically or philosophically to conduct such studies. In many cases they just do not have the time or staff assistance to conduct the analysis. A vicious cycle ensues where program changes cause problems that could have been avoided. A new change—equally understudied for financial consequences—is introduced, only aggravating the situation further.

As far as nurse administrators are concerned, the days of not being analytical in the face of significant program changes are certainly past. A commitment to predicting the financial impact of changes in nursing programs is clearly needed. This means that nurse administrators must undertake analysis in order to guide decision making. For example, consider the option of adding a day hospital in the acute care setting. The chief executive officer is promoting the concept because it will fill unused bed capacity. There will be more revenue where previously there was less. Should the nurse administrator lend support to such a concept? This question can best be answered analytically.

The nurse manager may complete the following analysis:

Addition of Proposed Day Care Hospital

Program Concept:

1. Allocate ten beds for day care.
2. Staff with emergency department physicians who allocate time as needed.
3. Add one full-time registered nurse on the day shift to provide nursing coverage.
4. Charge $42 per patient per day.
5. Forecast 90 percent occupancy in the first year's operation.

Feasibility Analysis:

Revenues	=	$42 per patient day × 10 beds × .9 occupancy × 365 days
	=	$42 × 10 × .9 × 365
	=	$137,970
Costs	=	nursing time + support services + physician supplement + rent for space
	=	$39,200 + $65,000 + 18,000 + 15,000
	=	$137,200
Net Revenue	=	$137,970 − $137,200 = $770

Should the nurse administrator support this proposal?

The financial analysis suggests that the program is marginal in its ability to return revenues to the hospital. However, consider the alternative. It offers greater occupancy from which total hospital economies of scale can be derived. It expands the services of the hospital and therefore the ability to market a full range of services. The medical staff, particularly the emergency room physicians, are pleased because income is supplemented. Moreover the presence of the day care program presents the prospect of patient referrals that the medical staff views as vital. The hospital has a new specialty that may grow and thereby increase the occupancy level. Furthermore, the image of the hospital as an innovator will improve.

But what about nursing? In this illustration there only appears to be a positive impact on nursing; is there? Examine the advantages and disadvantages from the nursing director's perspective:

Advantages:

1. Expands staff, thereby adding to the centrality of nursing services in the hospital.
2. Provides an opportunity for the nursing staff to specialize in an evolving clinic area such as gerontological nursing or rehabilitation.
3. Expands the hospital's program to attract more nurses who might help improve the skills of the total nursing staff.
4. Presents an opportunity to transfer patients from marginal inpatient status to ambulatory status yet maintain some control over their recuperation.

Disadvantages:

1. Requires an added staff member—recruiting is already difficult with several unfilled positions.
2. Opens a new clinical specialization, yet provides no convenient mechanism for integrating that specialization with existing services.
3. Proposes no mechanism for funding the additional administration of the program by the nursing department; the day care nurse must be supervised by the nursing department.
4. Includes no standards for the nurse's productivity or for quality of care.
5. Makes no guarantees for the intended level of occupancy; no contingency plans exist for use of the registered nurse if occupancy does not reach the intended level.
6. Requires the nurse to interface with the continuing education program for nursing, yet makes no allocations for this.

On balance, the proposed day care hospital is financially feasible for the hospital but there are some questions regarding the feasibility for the nursing program.

If the nursing director were exceptionally concerned about the program after considering the advantages and disadvantages, it might be appropriate to consider costing out the disadvantages noted above. This exercise is not intended to prove to hospital management that it has a very bad or good idea. The issue is to alert the administrator to the fact that the program feasibility study incorporates only explicit costs and revenues. From the nursing department's perspective there are many added costs, both real and psychic, that suggest uncertainty about the program. Remember that these costs are offset by advantages that have not been evaluated for their monetary contribution. The nursing director needs to use this information to either obtain more resources or to underscore the nursing department's position in obtaining budgetary supplements.

Suboptimizing Performance

Nurse administrators need to determine the appropriateness of suboptimizing performance when considering the strategies of financial management. It is paradoxical that less than perfect performance is often viewed as the best performance, but this may be true. Suboptimizing performance is particularly essential in large health care organizations confronting the constraints of prospective payment and competition. They need to derive the best performance possible from each work unit, program, or department. However, it is vital that the performance of the entire organization not suffer because of the best intentions of any single performer. In other words, programs may be asked to suboptimize their achievements in order to help achieve optimal organizational performance.

An illustration may help to demonstrate the concept of suboptimizing and why it is financially important. Consider the nursing department that is under pressure to hold down costs. In order to make its best contribution it begins to enforce two distinct strategies. On one hand it begins to concentrate only on delivering clinical services, and on the other hand it delivers care with small yet significant shortcuts in the treatment of patients. Over the course of the first year the hospital experiences lower costs and thereby a better operating margin. But has financial performance actually been improved?

From the surface it appears that the organization is performing better because of the lower costs. But nursing has suboptimized its interests to an excessive extent. By concentrating only on delivering clinical services it has failed to make a contribution to support programs that are valuable in providing outreach. Therefore the hospital may not attract consumers in the same manner as it has in the past. Eventually patient revenues are lost because these programs are not in place. Furthermore, by sanctioning shortcuts in the delivery of care that raise productivity but neglect the quality of care, the hospital may encounter more malpractice suits that severely cut into financial performance.

The lesson from this example should be clear. Maximization of financial performance over the short run can lead to poor financial performance in the long run. Although nursing programs and departments need to subordinate their interests in order to help the entire organization achieve its goals, it is also vital in so doing that they do not hamper the long-run financial performance.

THE NURSING ENTREPRENEUR

A final consideration that nursing managers need to ponder is the need to promote entrepreneurial activity. More than ever health care organizations need a vibrant entrepreneurial spirit among the staff that facilitates diversification and cements loyalty from consumers. The nurse manager can play an effective role in directing personnel toward this goal.

Nurses are in a pivotal position to address the pressures confronting health care organizations and therefore foster an entrepreneurial spirit for several reasons. First, there are very few health care services that are not based upon strong nursing services. Acute, chronic, and primary care all depend upon a strong system of nursing services. Acute care is most viable where nursing care assists patients in their recovery from acute illness. Physicians are vital to medical care, but nurses have the biggest impact on acute patient care. Chronic long-term care is essentially nurse dominated. There are few geriatricians or other providers oriented specifically to the elderly and long-term care patient. Nurses are usually the front line in caring for the long-term care patient. They have the education to intervene and they are close enough to the patient to monitor progress. Primary care appears to be physician dominated, but the growth of nurse specialists as mid-level professionals has allowed them to take an active role in primary care. Thus, from all aspects—acute, chronic, and primary care—nurses are the main professional support for the health care system.

Second, since nurses are responsible for delivery of services they also have an opportunity to control many of the costs associated with service delivery. Few would argue that physicians still retain control over medical care decisions. However, nurses control the many operational decisions surrounding the delivery of nursing and medical care. They have considerable ability to control the use of supplies, equipment, and support personnel in a health care organization. Here is where cost control can attain an entrepreneurial spirit in the health system. The ability to manage inputs into the delivery process provides nurses an exceptional opportunity to determine whether a health care organization is able to control costs innovatively.

Third, nurses know how organizations function. They understand the need to work within an organizational framework. Hence they are more likely to support creative team efforts to control costs, pursue quality of care, or strive for profitability. Organizations will play a dominant role in attaining high quality and cost-effective health care in the future. The growth of entrepreneurial health care corporations, particularly investor-owned corporations, is indicative of this shift in orientation. The health system will have to continue entrepreneurial efforts in order to attain high quality care at low cost. However, this entrepreneurial effort will be organizationally based (e.g., multi-institutional organizations) rather than individually based (e.g., freestanding hospitals or solo practitioners).

The preceding thoughts point to an inevitable conclusion. Nurses not only are in a position to improve the entrepreneurial management of health care organizations, they also possess associated education, attitudes, and values that can help them become key managers. Critical to the growth of nurse administrators is a firm understanding of financial management concepts. Whereas commitment to high quality of care used to drive the health care system, the reality is that resources are now constrained. Prospective pricing has had a substantial impact in motivating health care organizations to change their attitudes and methods of managing. Given a decrease in the pace of allowable rate increases and in some instances caps on further increases, health care organizations are facing troublesome revenue projections. Since revenues are being held relatively constant, the best opportunity to derive net profits is by controlling the costs associated with the delivery of services or production of goods. This is easy to say, but in reality someone must achieve the cost control. Nurse administrators are in valuable positions to make this sort of contribution.

THE NURSE ADMINISTRATOR AND FINANCIAL MANAGEMENT

Unless nurse administrators become proficient in financial management concepts and their application, it is unlikely that they will be able to take advantage of the managerial opportunities presented by competition and prospective payment. They must be capable of thinking, communicating, and supervising in financial terms if they expect to exploit and enjoy the opportunities. This means more than just becoming familiar with the technical aspects of financial management. It also means managing from the perspective of financial sensitivity. Hence nurse administrators need to adopt a financial perspective that they can implement not only in their work units, programs, or departments, but also in how they interact with other managers throughout the health care organization.

In sum, knowing how to rate capital investments by undertaking the required analysis (e.g., internal rate of return, payback, or net present value), establishing a budget that is consistent with organizational plans, obtaining financing to cover short-term or long-term capital needs, maximizing inflows from third party payers, assessing the status of an organization by reviewing financial statements and reports, evaluating performance in terms of ratios, or establishing a plan for managing working capital, are all important skills in financial management. Nurse administrators who acquire such knowledge are undoubtedly technically better prepared to complete the management requirements of their positions. However, skill application, alone, is not enough. Nurse administrators must integrate financial knowledge and skills into a philosophy of how health care organizations and nursing programs should operate. A nursing orientation should not dominate the management of a program or department. The nurse administrator must also address the financial needs of the health care organization.

NOTES

1. Aaron Levenstein, "Economic Hygiene for Hospitals," *Supervisor Nurse* 7 (October 1976): 88.
2. Muriel A. Poulin, "The Nurse Executive Role," *Journal of Nursing Administration* 14 (February 1984): 9–14.
3. Letty Roth Piper, "Managing the Intermediate Product," *Nursing Management* 16 (March 1985): 18–20.
4. William O. Cleverley, "How Much Profit Should a Hospital Make?" *Hospital Financial Management* 32 (January 1978): 22–28.
5. Floyd Kinkead, "An Economic Profit for Hospitals Is a Fiscal Fact of Life," *Hospital Financial Management* 30 (July 1976): 40–42.
6. Howard L. Smith and Nancy W. Mitry, "Nursing Leadership: A Buffering Perspective," *Nursing Administration Quarterly* (Spring 1984): 43–52.
7. Mary Ann Haw et al., "Improving Nursing Morale in a Climate of Cost Containment: Part 1. Organizational Assessment," *Journal of Nursing Administration* 14 (October 1984) 8–15.

Answers to Self Study Exercises

ANSWERS TO SELF STUDY EXERCISES IN CHAPTER 3

Liquidity Ratios

1. Current Ratio $= \dfrac{\text{Current Assets}}{\text{Current Liabilities}} = \dfrac{\$55,700}{\$140,000} = 0.40$

2. Acid Test Ratio $= \dfrac{\text{Current Assets} - \text{Inventory}}{\text{Current Liabilities}} = \dfrac{\$48,200}{\$140,000} = 0.34$

3. Days In Accounts Receivable $=$

$\dfrac{\text{Net Accounts Receivable} \times 365}{\text{Net Operating Revenue} \div 365} = \dfrac{\$44,200 \times 365}{\$28,424} = 567.6$

4. Average Payment Period $=$

$\dfrac{\text{Current Liabilities} \times 365}{\text{Total Operating Expenses} - \text{Depreciation}} = \dfrac{\$140,000 \times 365}{\$123,686 - \$100,000} = 2157.4$

Profitability Ratios

5. Return on Total Assets $= \dfrac{\text{Net Income}}{\text{Total Assets}} = \dfrac{\$30,000}{\$2,130,700} = 0.14$

6. Operating Margin $= \dfrac{\text{Operating Income}}{\text{Total Operating Revenue}} = \dfrac{\$28,424}{\$152,110} = 0.19$

Activity Ratios

7. $\text{Total Asset Turnover} = \dfrac{\text{Total Operating Revenue}}{\text{Total Assets}} = \dfrac{\$152,110}{\$2,130,700} = 0.07$

8. $\text{Current Asset Turnover} = \dfrac{\text{Total Operating Revenue}}{\text{Current Assets}} = \dfrac{\$152,110}{\$55,700} = 2.73$

Leverage Ratios

9. $\text{Debt to Total Assets} = \dfrac{\text{Total Debts}}{\text{Total Assets}} = \dfrac{\$1,930,700}{\$2,130,700} = 0.91$

10. $\text{Debt to Equity} = \dfrac{\text{Long-Term Debt}}{\text{Equity}} = \dfrac{\$1,790,700}{\$200,000} = 8.95$

Interpretation of Ratios

The liquidity ratios suggest that this organization is experiencing financial difficulties. The liquidity ratios indicate a low ratio of current assets to current debt. The days in accounts receivable and average payment period are excessively long. However, the profitability ratios indicate marginal performance in terms of the net income derived to total assets. A partial problem exists due to low asset turnover, as seen in the activity ratios. The primary problem is overleverage, as seen in the leverage ratios. There is too much debt to equity.

ANSWERS TO SELF STUDY EXERCISES IN CHAPTER 8

1. Compound interest factor for 12% at 5 years = 1.762
   Interest charged = (1.762 × $20,000) − $20,000 = $15,240
2. Present value = ($2,000)(.873) = $1,746
3. Annuity factor for 9% at 5 years = 3.890
   Present value = ($287,941)(3.890) = $1,120,090.40
4. *Payback Method:*
   Original investment = $5,000
   Super Bubbly requires 2 years ($3,000 + $2,500) to return the original investment
   Quiet Stream requires 3 years ($2,000 + $1,500 + $1,500) to return the original investment
   The nursing home should purchase the Super Bubbly

Present Worth Method:

Year	Interest Factor	Super Bubbly		Quiet Stream	
		12% Cost of Capital			
1	.893	× $3,000 =	$2,679	× $2,000 =	$1,786
2	.797	× 2,500 =	1,993	× 1,500 =	1,196
3	.712	× 500 =	356	× 1,500 =	1,068
4	.636			× 1,500 =	954
5	.567			× 500 =	284
	Present Worth =		$5,028		$5,288

The nursing home should purchase the Quiet Stream.

Summary Chart of Financial Ratios

Liquidity Ratios: these ratios measure the extent to which short-run obligations can be met by the organization

$$Current\ Ratio\ =\ \frac{Current\ Assets}{Current\ Liabilities}$$

$$Acid\ Test\ Ratio\ =\ \frac{Current\ Assets\ -\ Inventory}{Current\ Liabilities}$$

$$Days\ in\ Accounts\ Receivable\ =\ \frac{Net\ Accounts\ Receivable\ \times\ 365}{Net\ Operating\ Revenue}$$

$$Average\ Payment\ Period\ =\ \frac{Current\ Liabilities\ \times\ 365}{Total\ Operating\ Expenses\ -\ Depreciation}$$

$$Days\ Cash\ on\ Hand\ =\ \frac{(Marketable\ Securities\ +\ Cash)\ \times\ 365}{Total\ Operating\ Expenses\ -\ Depreciation}$$

Profitability Ratios: these ratios measure the level of net revenue or income relative to a given level of equity

$$Return\ on\ Equity\ (Fund\ Balance)\ =\ \frac{Net\ Income}{Fund\ Balance}$$

$$Return\ on\ Total\ Assets\ =\ \frac{Net\ Income}{Total\ Assets}$$

$$Operating\ Margin\ =\ \frac{Operating\ Income}{Total\ Operating\ Revenue}$$

$$Nonoperating\ Revenue\ Ratio\ =\ \frac{Nonoperating\ Revenue}{Net\ Income}$$

$$\textit{Discounts and Allowances Ratio} = \frac{\text{Discounts, Allowances, and Uncollectibles}}{\text{Patient Revenue}}$$

Activity Ratios: these ratios measure the extent to which an organization is efficiently using its assets

$$\textit{Total Asset Turnover} = \frac{\text{Nonoperating Revenue}}{\text{Net Income}}$$

$$\textit{Current Asset Turnover} = \frac{\text{Total Operating Revenue}}{\text{Current Assets}}$$

$$\textit{Fixed Asset Turnover} = \frac{\text{Total Operating Revenue}}{\text{Total Fixed Assets}}$$

$$\textit{Inventory Turnover} = \frac{\text{Total Operating Revenue}}{\text{Inventory}}$$

Leverage Ratios: these ratios assess the amount of debt relative to equity held by an organization

$$\textit{Debt Ratio} = \frac{\text{Total Debt}}{\text{Total Assets}}$$

$$\textit{Times Interest Earned} = \frac{\text{Earnings Before Interest and Taxes}}{\text{Interest}}$$

$$\textit{Debt to Equity} = \frac{\text{Long-Term Debt}}{\text{Equity}}$$

$$\textit{Total Assets to Equity} = \frac{\text{Total Assets}}{\text{Equity}}$$

Glossary of Terms

Accounts receivable: Payments owed to an economic enterprise due to services or products provided.

Accounts payable: Short-term debts incurred in the provision of services or products.

Accrual versus cash reporting: Accounting under which system a transaction is reported on financial statements only if it affects equity, even if there is no net effect on cash. The cash basis reports any alteration in cash, whether or not equity is affected.

Activity ratio: A measure of the extent to which an organization is efficiently using its assets.

Age of accounts: Number of days over which bills have not been paid.

Allowance for uncollectibles: Adjustments to accounts receivable that reflect the extent of free care or bad debts.

Annuities: Recurrent, periodic, equal-sized payments of money (e.g., monthly mortgage payments).

Asset: A resource with exchange or economic value.

Average rate of return: A method for calculating the return on an investment where the investment return is adjusted by the asset's economic life and actual expenditures during the life of the asset.

Balance sheet: A financial report that provides information on the status of assets, liabilities, and fund balances. This report profiles the economic condition of an organization.

Board-designated funds: Funds donated to an organization that can be used at the discretion of the board.

Bond: A legal contract where the issuer agrees to make specified interest payments and to repay borrowed principal at an agreed date of maturity.

Bond ratings: Independent assessments by financial organizations that assess the risk and yield of bonds.

Bond yield: The interest rate attached to a bond.

Budgeting: The implementation of plans. Budgeting is the tactical or operational element of the planning process.

Capital assets: Long-term assets such as facility, plant, and major pieces of equipment.

Capital budget: A periodic schedule for the disbursement of funds for capital expenditures.

Capital budgeting: The process of planning and decision making for capital assets including determining the need for additional assets, ascertaining the financial feasibility, evaluating asset options, and integrating capital expenditures within the long-run financial plans.

Cash flow budget: A plan for cash receipts and disbursements.

Compound interest: A method of calculating interest expense that recognizes the time value of money. Interest earned on interest.

Contractual allowances: Formal agreements between third party payers and providers for discounts or adjustments to the rate of reimbursement.

Control: The management process that identifies deviations in performance from either broad plans or specific budgets and corrects those deviances.

Cost of capital: The rate of return that must be earned on a capital investment to maintain the economic value of the health care institution.

Cost variance analysis: Analytical determination of how and why costs vary. Often undertaken by calculating standard costs that link goods or services with the precise resources consumed in their production.

Current asset: A resource that is in negotiable form or could be converted into negotiable form within a short period of time.

Decision support system: An information system that is oriented toward unstructured problems, uses combinations of models and analytical techniques, and emphasizes an interactive mode.

Depreciation: An allowable expense for tax purposes that represents the wear or deterioration experienced by an asset.

Direct costs: Costs that can be identified with and that result from the production of a specific good or delivery of a specific service.

Electronic data processing: An automated system that performs data storage, retrieval, and transaction processing.

Expert system: A computer system that applies artificial intelligence to solve difficult problems.

Financial lease: An agreement between a lessor and lessee for extended use of an asset. Mainly provides access to an asset, seldom with a covenant for service.

Financial management: The management of an organization's capital assets, revenues, and uses to achieve specific goals.

Fixed asset: A resource that is judged to have a long economic life.

Fixed costs: Costs that do not vary with the volume of goods or services produced (e.g., monthly mortgage cost).

Forecasting: A projection for operations such as demand, cost, or revenue.

Fund accounting: A method of categorizing funds on the balance sheet that explicitly addresses the use of these funds for special purposes. Donors may restrict their charitable contributions for special projects (e.g., construction of a building). Alternatively, the funds may be assigned to a specific endowment (e.g., allocated to continuing nursing education). These funds are reported separately from operating assets due to tax implications.

Indirect costs: Costs that cannot be directly traced to a specific good or service, even though the indirect cost may be necessary to produce the good or service.

Information system: A manual and/or computer-based system for information processing. Information is provided to management for purposes of planning and decision making.

Internal rate of return: A method for calculating the return on an investment that incorporates the time value of money—the rate that equates the present value of future returns with the initial investment.

Inventory: Supplies necessary to provide services or to produce products.

Lease: Acquisition of an asset without the transfer of ownership.

Leverage ratio: A measure of the amount of debt relative to equity held by an organization.

Liabilities: Financial responsibilities and debts resulting from current operations and investment in fixed assets.

Liquidity ratio: A measure of financial performance that indicates the extent to which short-run obligations can be met.

Long-term debt: Debt that will typically be repaid over a period greater than one year. This debt is usually acquired in obtaining fixed assets.

Marketable securities: Short-term investments that can be easily liquidated into cash.

Net income: The difference between revenues and expenses.

Net operating revenue: The balance of total operating revenues less total operating expenses.

Nonoperating revenue: Revenue that is derived from sources other than current operations, such as monetary donations, sale of assets, or donated assets.

Operating budget: A periodic schedule that estimates use, expenses, and revenues over a fiscal period.

Operating expenses: Expenses incurred when conducting business; that is, providing services or producing products.

Operating lease: A written contract for use of an asset where the lessor provides services (e.g., maintenance) relating to the asset.

Operating margin: The difference between operating revenues and operating expenses.

Other operating revenue: Revenue derived from operations that are not directly related to patient care.

Patient care revenues: Monies or revenue received in exchange for the delivery of services and products.

Payback method: A method of calculating the return on an investment that ascertains how many years are required to return the original investment.

Periodic interim payments: Periodic payments from third party payers that promote cash flow.

Planning: The management process that articulates specific end results to be achieved and the strategy for doing so. Strategic planning involves the major goals and objectives of an organization. Medium-range planning determines specific department, divisional, or program plans in order to allocate resources. Short-range planning incorporates budgeting to allocate resources during the fiscal period.

Portfolio: A set of investments by an individual or an organization.

Precollected revenue: Revenue collected before products or services are delivered.

Present value or present worth: The current value of a compounded sum of money.

Profitability ratio: A measure of financial performance that defines the extent of net revenue or income compared with a given level of equity.

Revenue adjustments: Changes made in gross revenues to reflect deductions such as allowances for charity, bad debts, and contractual allowances.

Risk: The probability that a variable or event will deviate from its expected value.

Semivariable costs: Costs that vary with volume, but at other times are fixed (e.g., equipment maintenance).

Statement of changes in fund balance: A financial report that provides information on how fund balances have changed over a fiscal period due to current operations, philanthropy, fund-raising, or other factors that influence fund balances.

Statement of revenues and expenses: A financial report that provides information on expenses, revenues, and net income. This report profiles the ability of an organization to keep expenses below revenues.

Step costs: Costs that remain fixed for various volume levels but increase by specific increments at certain volumes (e.g., total staff salaries increase by a major step every time a new staff member is hired).

Total operating revenue: Total patient care revenues and other operating revenues less deductions for discounts and allowances.

Trade credits: A favorable credit that can be received for prompt payment of current liabilities.

Uniform reporting: Standardized reporting formats used to record data for regulatory and reimbursement agencies.

Variable costs: Costs that vary with the volume of goods or services produced (e.g., medical supplies).

Working capital: Generally viewed as the current assets of an organization. However, current assets have meaning in relation to current liabilities. Hence, working capital is the difference between current assets and current liabilities.

Index

C

sale-and-leaseback, 225-226
Leverage ratios, 72-76, 282
  debt to equity (DTE) ratio, 75
  debt to total assets (DTA) ratio, 73-74
  times interest earned (TIE) ratio, 74
  total assets to equity (TAE) ratio, 75-76
Liabilities, 29
Liquidity ratios, 59-64, 281
  acid test ratio, 60-61
  average payment period (APP) ratio, 62-63
  current ratio, 60
  days in accounts receivable (DAR) ratio, 61-62
  days cash on hand (DCH) ratio, 63-64
Lock boxes, 168-169
Long-term assets, as capital assets, 201
Long-term debt, capital, source of, 242
Long-term operations, balanced with current
  operations, 152-155
Longitudinal analysis
  financial ratios, 76-79
    basic assumptions, 76-77
    as foundation for investigation, 77

M

Major diagnostic categories (MCDs), 6
Management information systems (MIS), 107-108
Market activity, as planning issue, 91-92
Marketable securities
  role of, 161-162
  types of, 161
Master budgets, 98-99, 113, 120
  capital budget, 98, 99, 120
  cash flow budget, 98, 99, 120
  operating budget, 98, 99, 120
Medicare
  Medicare Provider Analysis and Review (MEDPAR), 7

prospective pricing legislation, 6, 7
Medium-range planning, 89
  parameters of, 90
Multi-institutional systems, capital, source of, 241

N

Net income, 35
Net operating expenses, 34
  nonoperating expenses, 34
Network, HMO, 13
Nonprofit hospitals, compared to investor-owned hospitals, 9-11
Nonoperating revenue, sources of, 153
Nonoperating revenues (NOR) ratio, 67-68
Nonprofitability concept, 238-239
Nurse administrators role, 1-2, 265-275
  financial analysis, 270-273
  monitoring reimbursement trends, 266-269
  negotiation with top management, 270
  as nursing entrepreneur, 273-275
  suboptimizing performance, 273
  See also specific topics.
Nursing acuity, 197-199
Nursing budgets, 135-138
  decentralized, 145
Nursing costs, calculation by acuity, 197-199

O

Operating budget, 98, 99
Operating expenses, 34-35
Operating lease, 225
Operating margin, components of, 154-155
Operating margin (OM) ratio, 66
Operating performance report, 48-50
Operating revenue, sources of, 153

Regulation
  as planning issue, 94
  of reimbursement, 94
Reimbursement, and leasing, 227-228
Reimbursement trends, as planning
  issue, 93-94
Reporting data, uniform reporting, 47
Restricted funds, 23
Return on equity (ROE) ratio, 64, 65
Return on funds, planning of, 160-161
Return on total assets (ROA) ratio, 65-
  66
Revenue forecast, 126-130
  complexity of, 127
  components of, 127-128
  income statement and, 129-130
  support services and, 128-129
Revenue streams, 168-170
  lock boxes, 168-169
  per diem rate method, 169
  percentage of charges rate method,
    169
  periodic interim payments, 170
Revenues
  operating, 34
  patient care, 34
  total operating, 34

Standard cost system, 192-194
  example of, 193-194
  goal of, 192-193
  steps for, 192
Statement of changes in fund balances,
  36-40, 221
  balance sheet and, 37
  purpose of, 36
  terminology, changes in, 37
Statement of revenues and expenses
  compared to income statement, 32
  as management tool, 31-32
  nonprofit organizations, 30
  primary purposes of, 30-31
  terminology used, 34-35
  unmatched revenues/expenses, 35
Statistical forecast, 120-122
  elements of, 122
  techniques used, 121-122
Statistical performance report, 50
Stock offerings, 205-206
Straight-line method, 43
  unit costs, 183
Strategic planning, 89, 96-97
Subject models, 104
Sum-of-years-digits, 43-44

S

Sale-and-leaseback, 225-226
Secure cash handling
  factors involved, 159-160
  planning of, 159-160
Securities, marketable, 161-162
Semivariable costs, 185-187
Short-range planning, 89
  importance of, 90-91
Short-term debt, 171-173
  pitfalls to avoid, 172-173
  sources of, 171-172
Staff model, HMO, 13
Staff participation
  and control, 100-101
  eliciting participation, guidelines for,
    100-101

T

Tax Equity and Fiscal Responsibility
Act (TEFRA), 7
Tax-exempt revenue bonds
  capital, source of, 242-247
  features of, 243-2442
  ratings of, 244-247
    generic hospital characteristics and,
      247
    investment agency assessment,
      245-256
    rating firms, 245
Tax-exempt status, 10
Third party payment
  as planning issue, 93-94
  working capital management and,
    151-152